CPET Made Simple

CPET Made Simple

A Practical Guide to Cardiopulmonary Exercise Testing

Tom Lawson
Swansea Bay University Health Board

Helen Anderson
University Hospitals Plymouth NHS Trust

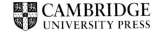
CAMBRIDGE
UNIVERSITY PRESS

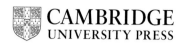

Shaftesbury Road, Cambridge CB2 8EA, United Kingdom

One Liberty Plaza, 20th Floor, New York, NY 10006, USA

477 Williamstown Road, Port Melbourne, VIC 3207, Australia

314–321, 3rd Floor, Plot 3, Splendor Forum, Jasola District Centre,
New Delhi – 110025, India

103 Penang Road, #05–06/07, Visioncrest Commercial, Singapore 238467

Cambridge University Press is part of Cambridge University Press & Assessment,
a department of the University of Cambridge.

We share the University's mission to contribute to society through the pursuit of
education, learning and research at the highest international levels of excellence.

www.cambridge.org
Information on this title: www.cambridge.org/9781009412889

DOI: 10.1017/9781009412896

First published 2024

A catalogue record for this publication is available from the British Library

Library of Congress Cataloging-in-Publication Data
Names: Lawson, Tom (Consultant anaesthetist), author. | Anderson, Helen (Consultant
anaesthetist), author.
Title: CPET made simple : a practical guide to cardiopulmonary exercise testing / Tom Lawson,
Helen Anderson.
Description: Cambridge, United Kingdom ; New York, NY : Cambridge University Press, 2024. |
Includes bibliographical references and index.
Identifiers: LCCN 2023041918 | ISBN 9781009412889 (paperback) | ISBN 9781009412896
(ebook)
Subjects: MESH: Exercise Test – methods | Exercise – physiology
Classification: LCC RM725 | NLM WG 141.5.F9 | DDC 615.8/2–dc23/eng/20231208
LC record available at https://lccn.loc.gov/2023041918

ISBN 978-1-009-41288-9 Paperback

Contents

Contents

Glossary

- **Anaerobic Threshold (AT)** – the point beyond which oxygen demand exceeds the supply from aerobic metabolism alone and is supplemented by anaerobic metabolism.

- **ATPS** – ambient temperature, pressure, saturated with water (units used on some CPET plots).

- **Breathing Reserve (BR)** – the difference between maximum voluntary ventilation (MVV) and maximum exercise ventilation (VE). That is, BR = MVV – VE.

- **BTPS** – body temperature, pressure, saturated with water (units used on some CPET plots).

- **End-Tidal Partial Pressure of Carbon Dioxide/Oxygen (ETCO$_2$/ETO$_2$)** – partial pressure (mmHg) of exhaled CO_2 or O_2.

- **Ergometer** – a device that is used to quantify physical performance by providing a known workload.

- **Heart Rate Reserve (HRR)** – the difference between predicted and observed maximum heart rate during a cardiopulmonary exercise test.

- **Inspiratory Capacity** – volume of gas that can be maximally inhaled after a normal tidal exhalation.

- **Maximum Voluntary Ventilation (MVV)** – maximal volume of air that can be breathed per minute by a patient.

- **Oxygen Pulse (VO$_2$/HR)** – the oxygen uptake by pulmonary blood per heartbeat in ml/beat.

- **Respiratory Compensation Point (RCP)** – the point beyond which there is respiratory compensation for metabolic acidaemia, by increased ventilation.

- **Respiratory Exchange Ratio (RER)** – ratio of CO_2 production to O_2 consumption measured in expired gas. It reflects the metabolic exchange of gases in body tissues.

- **Respiratory Quotient (RQ)** – a dimensionless number that is calculated from the ratio of CO_2 production to O_2 consumption and is dictated by metabolic substrate.

- **STPD** – standard temperature, pressure, dry (units used on some CPET plots).

- **VCO_2** – the volume of CO_2 exhaled per unit time (ml/min).

- **VD/VT (Dead Space Fraction)** – the proportion of tidal volume that is made up of physiologic dead space. An index of V/Q mismatch.

- **VE** – minute ventilation (l/min), that is, the volume of gas that is exhaled in one minute.

- **Ventilatory Equivalents** – the volume of ventilation required to either take up a volume of oxygen ($VEVO_2$) or eliminate a volume of carbon dioxide ($VEVCO_2$).

- **Vital Capacity** – maximal volume of gas exhaled from the point of maximal inspiration.

- **VO_2** – oxygen consumption, that is, the volume of oxygen taken up from lungs to blood per unit time (ml/min).

- **VO_2 Max** – the maximum attainable oxygen uptake in ml/min for that individual.

- **VO_2 Peak** – the peak volume of oxygen uptake in ml/min for a particular test.

- **VO_2/Work Rate ($\Delta VO_2/\Delta WR$)** – increase in O_2 uptake in response to an increase in work rate – used to estimate the efficiency of muscular work.

- **Work** – the result of a force that causes movement or displacement of an object, defined by the formula, Work = force × distance (measured in kg/m).

- **Workload** – the external work (watts) that a patient exerts against the resistance of the ergometer.

- **Work Rate** – the rate at which work is done, that is, work per unit time – kg/m/min = watt.

Abbreviations

AT – anaerobic threshold
ATP – adenosine triphosphate
ATPS – ambient temperature, pressure, saturated with water
Bf – breathing frequency
bpm – beats per minute
BR – breathing reserve
BSA – body surface area
BTPS – body temperature, pressure, saturated with water
CaO_2 – arterial oxygen content
cm – centimetre
CO – cardiac output
CO_2 – carbon dioxide
COPD – chronic obstructive pulmonary disease
CPET – cardiopulmonary exercise test
CvO_2 – mixed venous oxygen content
CXR – chest X-ray
ECG – electrocardiogram
FEV_1 – forced expiratory volume in 1 second
FVC – forced vital capacity
H^+ – hydrogen ion(s)
$H_2CO_3^-$ – carbonic acid
H_2O – water
Hb – haemoglobin
HCO_3^- – bicarbonate
HR – heart rate
kg – kilogram
kPa – kilopascal
l – litre
m – metre
MET – metabolic equivalent
min – minute
ml – millilitre
mmHg – millimetres of mercury
MVV – maximum voluntary ventilation
O_2 – oxygen
OUES – oxygen uptake efficiency slope
$P(A-a)O_2$ – alveolar to arterial partial pressure gradient for oxygen
$PaCO_2$ – arterial partial pressure of carbon dioxide
PaO_2 – arterial partial pressure of oxygen
PEFR – peak expiratory flow rate

$PETCO_2$ – end-tidal partial pressure of carbon dioxide
$PETO_2$ – end-tidal partial pressure of oxygen
PO_2 – partial pressure of oxygen
Q – flow
QO_2 – total body oxygen delivery
RCP – respiratory compensation point
RER – respiratory exchange ratio
RQ – respiratory quotient
RR – respiratory rate
RV – residual volume
s – second
SaO_2 – arterial oxygen saturation
SpO_2 – peripheral oxygen saturation
SV – stroke volume
SvO_2 – venous oxygen saturation
TLC – total lung capacity
V – lung ventilation
VCO_2 – carbon dioxide production
Vd – dead space volume
VE – minute ventilation
$VEVCO_2$ – ventilatory equivalents for carbon dioxide
$VEVO_2$ – ventilatory equivalents for oxygen
VO_2 – oxygen consumption
Vt – tidal volume
W – watt
WR – work rate

Introduction

Cardiopulmonary exercise testing (CPET) has come a long way from its clinical introduction in the 1980s. It is a dynamic and integrative test that can assess cardiovascular, respiratory, skeletal muscular and metabolic responses to increasing exercise intensity. Such an investigation can be incredibly useful in the holistic assessment of a patient's functional status. It is no surprise then that this investigation is being increasingly used by cardiologists, respiratory physicians, exercise physicians, peri-operative physicians, anaesthetists, and physiologists for such diverse purposes as:

- Assessment of exercise capacity (and response to training, medication, etc.)
- Assessment of peri-operative risk
- Investigation, assessment, and prognostication in cardiac or respiratory disease
- Evaluation of endurance and performance in elite athletes.

Most of the current texts on this topic are extensive, looking into exercise physiology in-depth. As peri-operative physicians, we run holistic CPET clinics that receive referrals from all comers. The purpose of this book is to provide a concise introduction to cardiopulmonary exercise tests and their interpretation for their two most common in-hospital uses:

- Assessment of exercise capacity and peri-operative risk stratification
- Assessment of breathlessness.

Part I of this book will outline the basics of exercise physiology in the context of exercise testing.

Part II will examine the fundamentals for performing an exercise test, including indications/contraindications, safety, consent, equipment, ergometry, and test phases.

Part III discusses the key variables of and an approach to interpretation of a standard 9-panel plot of an exercise test.

Part IV will examine the use of CPET in assessment of exercise capacity (in the context of peri-operative risk stratification), assessment of dyspnoea, and any additional plots. There will be different case studies showing how the information from previous parts can be integrated together to form a comprehensive assessment.

We will not be covering the integration of invasive measurements into CPETs (this is beyond the scope of this text). Additionally, we will not cover other means of investigating exercise capacity, for example shuttle walk tests.

We hope this book will help to demystify and encourage clinicians to learn more about this valuable investigation, which can aid in the management of our patients.

| Chapter | # What Is Cardiopulmonary Exercise Testing? |
| 1 | |

Cardiopulmonary exercise testing (CPET) is a dynamic and objective investigation that studies the responses of the cardiovascular, respiratory, and skeletal muscular systems to exercise stress in an integrated way.

This is achieved by the measuring gas exchange, respiratory rate and volume, heart rate and ECG parameters, BP, and oxygen saturation (Figure 1.1) whilst a patient undertakes exercise using an ergometer (a device that is used to quantify physical performance by providing a known workload).

By simultaneously measuring cardiovascular and gas exchange parameters, we can relate them to actual energy expenditure during exercise and:

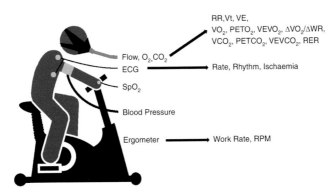

Figure 1.1 The typical set-up for a cardiopulmonary exercise test, different monitors and the measured/derived variables

- Assess functional status
- Identify and examine the underlying mechanisms that lead to exercise limitation and quantify the extent of limitation
- Investigate dyspnoea of unclear origin
- Detect and measure response to exercise, intervention, treatment, and/or pre- or rehabilitation
- Prognosticate on specific disease processes.

Why Perform a CPET?

The beauty of a CPET is its dynamic nature. It is a test performed with a patient that is moving, under strain. The limitation of many other investigations is their static nature, being performed with patients sitting down or lying on a bed, that is not under the same stress that exacerbates their symptoms. It is also an integrative test, looking at the functional integration of all of the components of the oxygen cascade, not just the heart and lungs independently like other dynamic tests, for example dobutamine stress ECHO or lung function tests. This makes the argument for its use in the assessment of cardiac or respiratory disease easy to comprehend.

In terms of its use as a tool in peri-operative risk stratification, it is useful to understand that major surgery is associated with a profound inflammatory response that can generate a significant increase in oxygen demand. Such surgery is associated with morbidity and mortality, especially in elderly patients and those with multiple or significant co-morbidities who may have reduced oxygen delivery with increased oxygen consumption.

Hence, a test that somewhat mimics the surgical stress response is desirable, and can be used to:

- Identify and stratify peri-operative risk
- Diagnose or quantify the impact of pre-existing conditions
- Modify peri-operative management
- Inform shared decision-making
- Provide a frame of reference for change with intervention or prehabilitation.

Chapter 2

Exercise Physiology

What Is Exercise?

- Exercise is any physical activity at a higher intensity than that of usual daily activity.
- Muscular activity (which can be defined in terms of external work rate or power output) results in an increase in energy demand, which is tightly coupled to oxygen demand, which is met by the ventilatory and circulatory systems.
- The physiological response to exercise (represented in Figure 2.1) involves a complex interrelation of various components, the extent of which depends on several factors, including duration and intensity of activity.

Work and Cellular Respiration

- Work is the result or product of a force that causes 'displacement' in the direction of the applied force (or energy transfer from one object to another):
  - Force = Mass × Acceleration,
  - Work = Force × Distance.
- Physiologically, we can divide work into the following two forms:
  - External work – the work done as muscular activity in order to move external objects
  - Internal work – all other forms of work, which are transferred as heat energy.
- In order to understand the fundamentals of cardiopulmonary exercise testing and how we might assess the functional capacity of the cardiorespiratory system, we need to examine the different physiological processes that couple external work and cellular respiration.

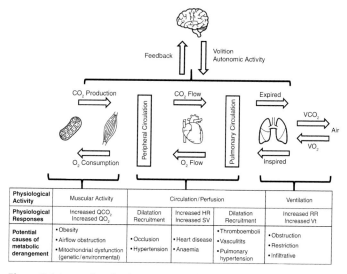

Figure 2.1 Interaction of various systems in the exercise response – adapted with permission from *Wasserman & Whipp's Principles of Exercise Testing and Interpretation: Including Pathophysiology and Clinical Applications*, sixth edition, Wolters Kluwer

- Chief amongst these measurements and estimations are:
  - Cardiac output
  - Minute ventilation
  - Respiratory gas composition.

Energy, Work, and ATP

Energy is needed to perform the work required while exercising. This energy is supplied via cellular metabolism. In simple terms, the food that we eat supplies us with the necessary substrate for energy production. During this process, energy is 'trapped' in molecules of adenosine triphosphate (ATP).

- This is the substance that is used for storage of energy and as a 'fuel' or energy 'currency' for cellular processes.
- A molecule of ATP is composed of adenine (a nitrogenous base), ribose (a five-carbon sugar), and a chain of three phosphates.

- Potential energy is stored in ATP by way of these three negatively charged, adjacent phosphate groups and their 'high-energy' phosphoanhydride bonds.
- When one of these bonds is broken by hydrolysis, the result is the formation of adenosine diphosphate (ADP) and the release of an inorganic phosphate (P_i) and energy:
  - $ATP + H_2O \leftrightarrow ADP + P_i + energy$.
- We use the term Gibbs free energy (G) to describe how energy changes within biochemical reactions.
- The change in free energy (ΔG) takes into account enthalpy (energy release or absorption) and entropy and determines whether a biochemical reaction is 'favourable', that is whether a reaction 'goes forward or not'.
- It is also influenced by
  - the properties/concentrations of the reactants
  - the environmental conditions of the reaction.
- Most reactions are reversible, and equilibrium is possible.
- We take the following simplified reaction, for example:
  - $A \leftrightarrow B$
    - If $\Delta G = 0$, the reaction is at equilibrium and does not proceed in favour of either direction.
    - If $\Delta G < 0$ (i.e. these are spontaneous reactions, no additional energy is required, and, as a result, free energy falls), the reaction favours $A \rightarrow B$.
    - If $\Delta G > 0$ (i.e. additional energy is required), the reaction favours $B \rightarrow A$.
- ΔG is sometimes expressed as $\Delta G°$ in terms of 'standard conditions' – 1 M of reactants and 1 atmosphere of pressure.
- Hydrolysis of ATP is accompanied by a reduction in free energy, the $\Delta G°$ being −7.3 kcal/mol.
- However, the intracellular concentrations of ATP are significantly higher than 1 M, such that the ΔG within a cell is approximately −12 kcal/mol.
- This means that ATP hydrolysis can be used to drive other energy-requiring cellular reactions, such as glycolysis.

Muscle contraction cannot occur without ATP, which, in addition to acting as an energy source, is used to fulfil the following functions:

- The generation of a muscle force by formation of actin–myosin cross-bridges.
- The use of Ca^{2+} as an intracellular messenger for muscle contraction by active transport of Ca^{2+} (but also Na^+ and K^+).

Metabolism and ATP Generation

- Metabolism is a series of biochemical reactions by which substrates absorbed after digestion are used to extract chemical energy, synthesise substances for structural maintenance and growth, and synthesise or detoxify waste products.
- There are three interlinked pathways based on fuel type: carbohydrate, protein, or lipid (Figure 2.2).
- There are several different mechanisms by which ATP can be generated, all of which predominately occur in mitochondria, and may depend on the presence of oxygen. They include:
  - Aerobic cellular respiration
  - Beta-oxidation of fatty acids (the shortening of fatty acid chains to produce acetyl-CoA)
  - Ketosis (the catabolism of ketone bodies)
  - Anaerobic cellular respiration.
- The presence of oxygen is of utmost importance in carbohydrate metabolism (the chief fuel substrate for exercise).
- In this process, one molecule of glucose is broken down into two molecules of pyruvate, which are then converted to acetyl-CoA, which enters the Krebs cycle (sometimes referred to as the citric or tricarboxylic acid cycle).
- A molecule of acetyl-CoA that completes one cycle (or 'turn') of the Krebs cycle will yield:
  - One ATP
  - Three NADH
  - One $FADH_2$
  - Two CO_2.
- H_2O is both produced and utilised during the Krebs cycle.
- NADH and $FADH_2$ are electron carriers. They are able to 'donate' electrons (NADH to a greater degree than $FADH_2$) via redox reactions as part of oxidative phosphorylation (also known as 'the electron transport chain').

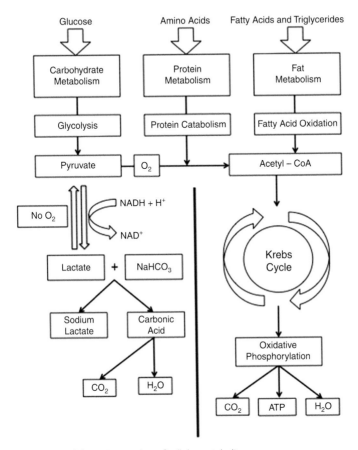

Figure 2.2 Schematic overview of cellular metabolism

- Electrons travel via mobile electron carriers along the inner mitochondrial membrane. In doing so, they release energy, which is utilised by various complexes to pump H^+ ions into the inter-membrane space.
- H^+ ions can then move down an electrochemical gradient back across the inner membrane via a trans-membrane protein: ATP synthase, which in turn catalyses the phosphorylation of ADP to ATP, in a process called chemiosmosis.

- The number of ATP molecules generated varies depending on the number of H^+ ions that can be generated, the efficiency of H^+ pumping, and so on.
- It is estimated that approximately 2–3 ATP molecules are generated per NADH and 1.5 molecules per $FADH_2$.
- The result is the generation of around 32–34 molecules of ATP (this is the most efficient system for ATP generation).

In the absence of oxygen, pyruvate is converted to lactate, generating a net of two ATPs. We will cover anaerobic respiration and lactate in more detail in the section titled 'Lactate and the Anaerobic Threshold'.

Muscle Cell Metabolism and ATP Source

During any form of exercise, there is an increase in muscular activity and cellular respiration in order to produce the ATP necessary for actin–myosin cross-bridging in individual muscle fibres. The location and source of ATP generation or utilisation depend on the intensity and duration of exercise. We can broadly think of exercise in two categories:
- Short duration
- Long duration.

Short Duration

- This form of exercise utilises the following energy sources:
  - ATP stored in muscles (which is depleted within 1 or 2 seconds)
  - Creatine phosphate, the breakdown of which is used to rapidly resynthesise ATP (this can fuel high-intensity efforts for approximately 10 seconds)
  - Anaerobic glycolysis (the breaking down of glycogen stored in muscles, which produces lactic acid as a by-product).

Long Duration

- The energy source utilised during longer durations of exercise depends on whether or not the anaerobic threshold (AT) has been reached.
- During steady-state exercise (below the AT), there is predominantly aerobic glycolysis, which feeds into the Krebs cycle and oxidative phosphorylation (initially using carbohydrate stores before moving on to fat with increased duration).

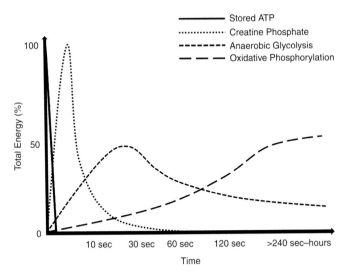

Figure 2.3 How energy source varies with exercise duration

- During non-steady-state exercise (beyond the AT), aerobic glycolysis continues – but it is not sufficient alone to meet cellular needs. Supplementation occurs by increasing anaerobic glycolysis, in which pyruvate is converted to lactate.

The interaction between energy source and exercise duration is shown in Figure 2.3.

Oxygen and Work

- Increased muscular activity increases O_2 demand and consumption (VO_2).
- Oxygen consumption (or uptake) is a measure of the body's ability to take in oxygen and deliver it to peripheral tissues via the cardiorespiratory system.
- VO_2 is determined by:
  - Cellular O_2 demand
  - O_2 extraction
  - O_2 transport.
- It is worth considering the anatomical structures that oxygen passes through and physiological processes involved in O_2

transport and extraction in order to understand the potential causes of limitation.

○ Oxygenation – the fraction of inspired O_2 relative to cellular demand
○ Ventilation – the process by which respiratory gases are transported from the outside world to the alveolar membrane (can be affected by airway patency and the bellows function of the lungs)
○ Diffusion – the process by which substances cross the alveolar–capillary interface (may be affected by factors such as concentration gradient and the thickness of the alveolar membrane)
○ Perfusion – the process by which adequate blood flow to the pulmonary capillaries is provided for gas exchange
○ Oxygen carriage in the blood (e.g. Hb level and factors affecting the Oxy–Hb dissociation curve)
○ Cardiac function
○ Peripheral blood flow – to supply muscles with oxygenated blood, and so on
○ Tissue perfusion (e.g. capillary density)
○ Tissue diffusion (i.e. diffusion of O_2 and CO_2 within tissue)
○ Mitochondrial density and function.

• The oxygen cost depends on work rate and duration.
We also need to introduce a few concepts (shown in Figure 2.4):
• O_2 deficit
○ This is the difference between an ideal hypothetical oxygen uptake and the actual oxygen uptake.
○ It represents a transient metabolic state in which additional energy is supplied by anaerobic processes until oxygen transport can meet the increased energy demand by normal means.
• O_2 debt
○ It is sometimes referred to as excess post-exercise oxygen consumption (EPOC).
○ It represents the state in which VO_2 remains elevated compared to pre-exercise levels.
○ This is the amount of oxygen required to restore the body to the pre-exercise state.
○ The ability to 'repay the debt' can be used as a means of evaluating cardiac function.

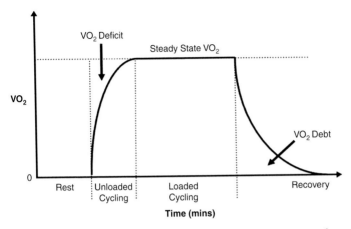

Figure 2.4 The relationship between oxygen consumption and duration of exercise

- Steady-state exercise – in essence, this is a stable state where VO_2 remains constant; CO_2 is only produced by metabolism and has a constant rate of elimination.
- Non-steady-state exercise – this is the exercise state above the anaerobic/lactate/ventilatory threshold where there is acidaemia and carotid body stimulation leading to a disproportionate rise in minute ventilation with increasing VO_2 (not shown in Figure 2.4).

VO_2–Work Rate Relationship

- Under normal circumstances, VO_2 increases in a linear fashion as external work increases.
- This shows that there is an efficient relationship between the body's metabolic ability to convert and utilise chemical energy and the ability of the musculoskeletal system to match the need for increased mechanical work.
- A failure of VO_2 to increase with increasing work rate implies inefficiency. We will discuss this in more detail in Part III.

Peak VO$_2$ and Max VO$_2$

- These terms are occasionally used interchangeably, and whilst it is possible that they may be the same, there is a distinct difference between peak VO$_2$ and max VO$_2$.
  - Peak VO$_2$
    - Peak VO$_2$ is achieved in a particular exercise test (Figure 2.5).
    - This is seen when VO$_2$ peaks and a test is terminated due to fatigue, and so on.
  - Max VO$_2$
    - The maximum VO$_2$ attainable by an individual (Figure 2.6) in that VO$_2$ cannot increase any further (or can only do so by a trivial amount). This is seen at peak exercise when maximal HR and SV are achieved, meaning that cardiac output cannot increase further, resulting in a VO$_2$ work rate plateau.

Lactate and the Anaerobic Threshold

- Glucose is the primary source of energy or fuel during exercise, and it undergoes glycolysis to form molecules of pyruvate.

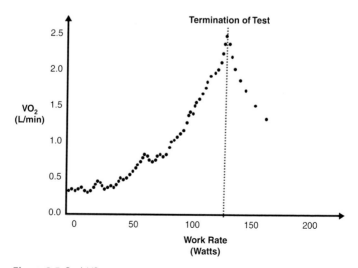

Figure 2.5 Peak VO$_2$

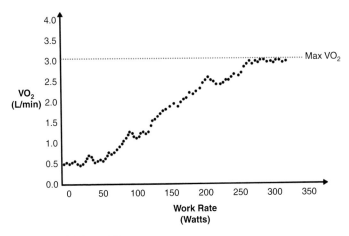

Figure 2.6 Maximum VO$_2$

- What then happens to pyruvate depends on the presence of oxygen, leading to either aerobic metabolism (pyruvate enters the Krebs cycle) or anaerobic metabolism (conversion to lactate).
- The rate of pyruvate formation versus the rate of oxidation depends on pyruvate dehydrogenase activity, the presence of oxygen, and mitochondrial oxidative capacity.
  - Under normal circumstances, exercise induces increased pyruvate dehydrogenase activity.
  - Activity is reduced by low oxygen and impaired mitochondrial oxidative capacity.
- Under anaerobic conditions, pyruvate is converted by lactate dehydrogenase to lactate (lactic acid).
- Additionally, if pyruvate formation exceeds oxidation to acetyl-CoA, there will be an increase in lactate production and accumulation.
- The production of lactate in relation to the metabolism of glucose and the Krebs (citric/tricarboxylic acid) cycle is shown in Figure 2.7.
- The level of lactate seen in blood depends on a number of factors:
  - The balance between lactate production and disposal
  - Level of exercise
  - Whether the sampled blood is arterial or venous.

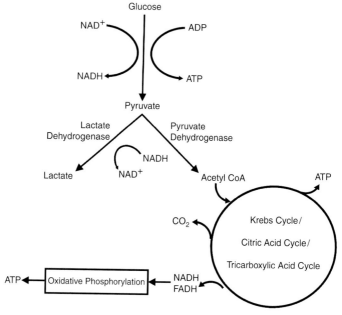

Figure 2.7 Glucose metabolism and lactate formation

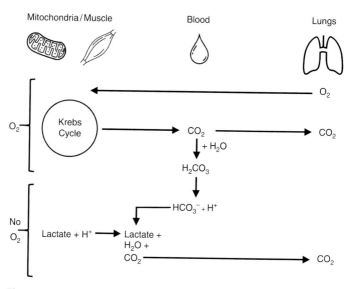

Figure 2.8 Lactic acid buffering

- A small increase in blood lactate will be seen even with low-intensity exercise but will usually stabilise.
- With higher exercise intensity, there is an accumulation of lactate (i.e. an imbalance between production and removal).
- The increase in lactic acid production (or rather the increase in H^+ ions from lactic acid) is buffered by HCO_3^- (shown in Figure 2.8).
  - $H^+ + HCO_3^- \leftrightarrow H_2CO_3 \leftrightarrow H_2O + CO_2$.
- This is what accounts for the increase in CO_2 seen at the AT.

Anaerobic Threshold, Ventilatory, and Cardiovascular Response to Exercise and the Fick Principle

- The term 'anaerobic threshold' (AT) can be tricky to define, and may vary depending on the discipline using it and the method of measurement.
- The AT can be measured in two ways during exercise testing:
  - Lactate AT (shown in Figure 3.1)
    - In this method, the AT is measured by taking sequential blood lactate levels.

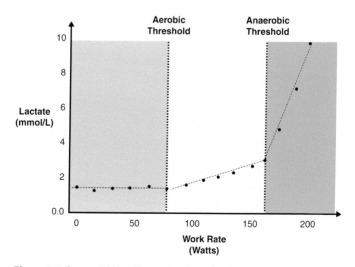

Figure 3.1 Sequential blood lactate levels used in determining the lactate AT

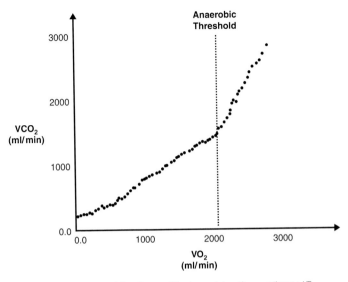

Figure 3.2 VCO_2 versus VO_2 plot used in determining the ventilatory AT

- Ventilatory AT (shown in Figure 3.2)
  - In this method, the AT is measured by respiratory gas analysis.
  - This is the point on a plot of VCO_2 versus VO_2 at which the VCO_2 increases more than VO_2.
  - This increase in CO_2 production is dealt with by an increase in ventilation.
- At low levels of exercise, whilst aerobic metabolism vastly predominates, there will be a degree of anaerobic metabolism (and as such, anaerobic pathways do not contribute a great deal to energy transfer).
- As exercise intensity increases, the proportion of anaerobic supplementation increases. The point at which this results in an increase in blood lactate level above a stable baseline is sometimes termed the 'aerobic threshold'.
- With increasing exercise intensity, a point will come at which lactate accumulation exceeds lactate removal, and blood lactate levels will increase further (associated with a reduction in

bicarbonate concentration and increase in CO_2 production as part of the buffering mechanism) – it is this point that is termed the AT.

- In terms of CPET, it is the ventilatory AT that we concern ourselves with. We shall examine the graphical representation of this concept later.

Ventilatory and Cardiovascular Response to Exercise

- Blood flow to musculature drastically increases by dilatation of selected peripheral vascular beds and increasing cardiac output (SV and HR) – shown in Figure 3.3.
- The increase in cardiac output is accompanied by an increase in pulmonary blood flow by recruitment and dilation of pulmonary blood vessels.
- There is an immediate initial increase in ventilation with the onset of exercise, followed by a slower exponential rise until a steady state is reached (shown in Figure 3.4). However, once the AT has been reached, ventilation will increase until either the cessation of exercise or exhaustion.
- Oxygen is taken up from the alveoli in proportion to the pulmonary blood flow and the degree of O_2 desaturation of Hb in pulmonary capillary blood.
- At steady state (at work rates below AT), $VO_2 = QO_2$.
  - QO_2 = total body oxygen delivery
- Meanwhile, ventilation (the product of tidal volume and respiratory rate) increases in relation to the newly produced CO_2 arriving at the lungs to maintain arterial CO_2 and H^+ ion homeostasis.

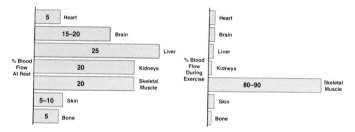

Figure 3.3 Blood flow changes in various vascular beds in response to exercise

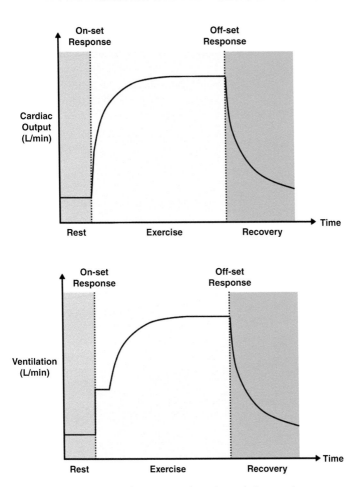

Figure 3.4 Changes in cardiac output and ventilation during exercise

The Fick Principle

The Fick principle (first described by Adolf Eugen Fick in 1870) is one of the key physiological concepts that underpins cardiopulmonary exercise testing. In his work, Fick described the use of oxygen as a 'marker substance' that could be used to measure the cardiac output of a dog's heart. In simple terms, the principle states:

- Arterial blood carrying oxygen flows through an organ.
- The organ will 'consume' oxygen from the blood.
- This will result in lower oxygen content in the blood leaving the organ.
  - This is the arterio-venous difference (measured in terms of volume of oxygen per unit volume of blood, for example millilitre per litre).
- If we know the total oxygen consumed by an organ, we can calculate the blood flow to that organ (see Figure 3.5) as

$$VO_2 = [\dot{Q} \times CaO_2] - [\dot{Q} \times C_vO_2].$$

- We can apply this to the whole body by substituting cardiac output (CO) for flow ($\dot{Q}$):

$$VO_2 = [CO \times CaO_2] - [CO \times C_vO_2],$$

which can be rearranged to

$$CO = VO_2/[CaO_2 - C_vO_2],$$

where

- CO = cardiac output
- VO_2 = oxygen consumption
- CaO_2 = arterial oxygen content
  - $CaO_2 = 1.34 \times Hb \times SaO_2 + (0.0031 \times PaO_2)$
- CvO_2 = mixed venous oxygen content.

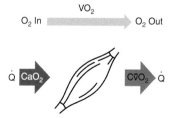

Figure 3.5 Representation of processes involved in the Fick principle

This is can be measured directly (e.g. by thermodilution), but in terms of cardiopulmonary exercise testing is measured indirectly via respiratory gas monitoring (in this scenario CO_2 is used as the marker substance):

- $CO = VCO_2/[CvCO_2 - CaCO_2]$,

  where

  - CO = cardiac output (L/min)
  - VCO_2 = CO_2 production (mL/min) – measured
  - $CvCO_2$ = venous carbon dioxide content – via CO_2 rebreathing
  - $CaCO_2$ = arterial carbon dioxide content – estimated from $PETCO_2$
- In this instance, the veno-arterial difference is used.
- It should be noted that there are many potential sources of error in this method and it is not considered to be wholly reliable.

Additionally, the Fick principle can be used to produce an indirect estimate of stroke volume (SV).

- During CPET, the variation of VO_2 with HR (the oxygen pulse) is measured.
- As we know cardiac output is the product of HR and SV,
  - $CO = SV \times HR$.
- We can therefore combine the oxygen pulse, together with the previous formula and the Fick principle, to show how the oxygen pulse can be used as an estimation of SV (covered in more detail in Part III).
  - $CO = VO_2/[CaO_2 - CvO_2]$,

  where $CaO_2 = 1.34 \times Hb \times SaO_2 + (0.0031 \times PaO_2)$.

  - Rearrange to:

    $VO_2 = CO \times [CaO_2 - CvO_2]$

  - Hence

    $VO_2 = [SV \times HR] \times [CaO_2 - CvO_2]$

  - If we assume the arteriovenous difference $(CaO_2 - CvO_2)$ to remain relatively constant, we can rearrange to:

$$\text{VO}_2/\text{HR} \approx \text{SV} = \text{O}_2 \text{ pulse}.$$

- Additionally, from these principles we can also see how a reduction in cardiac output results in reduced VO_2, and how various disease processes can affect each parameter, for example:
  - SV influenced by heart disease
  - HR influenced by heart disease, lung disease, muscle disease, and deconditioning
  - $[\text{CaO}_2 - \text{CvO}_2]$ influenced by anaemia, lung disease, mitochondrial function, oxygen extraction, and so on.
- This is of particular interest when we start examining each of the differing CPET plots.

Conduct of a CPET

CPET Safety, Indications, and Contraindications

CPET was initially used in the 1980s as a means of evaluating heart failure. In subsequent decades, its utility has been shown for a variety of indications across a wide variety of specialities. Indications include the following:

- Assessment of exercise capacity and development of training regimens
- Pre-op evaluation and risk stratification (this is the predominant reason in peri-operative practice)
- Evaluation of dyspnoea
  - Distinguishing cardiac versus pulmonary versus peripheral limitation versus other
  - Detection of exercise-induced bronchoconstriction
  - Detection of exertional desaturation
- Pulmonary rehabilitation
  - Exercise intensity/prescription
  - Response to participation in rehabilitation programmes
- Others
  - Diagnosis
  - Assessment of response to therapy
  - Prognostication of life expectancy
  - Disability determination.

In normal, healthy subjects, CPET is a relatively safe investigation. In non-healthy subjects (typically those with pre-existing cardiac disease), there are potential risks and CPET has been associated with morbidity and even mortality.

The incidence of such events is rare:

- Complication requiring hospitalisation – ≤2 per 1,000 tests

- Major cardiac event – 1.2 per 10,000 tests
- Death – two to five per 100,000 tests.

Therefore, it is important to understand the scenarios in which CPET would be contraindicated – these are outlined in Table 4.1 with relevant limits and time scales.

CPET and Complications

Whilst in general CPET is considered a safe investigation, it does put the body under increasing stress, and complications can occur (as outlined in the previous section). Hence the importance of adequate monitoring, access to resuscitation equipment, and trained staff for supervision. We can categorise common complications as follows:

- Cardiovascular
  - ECG changes (with or without anginal pain)
  - Blood pressure related changes
- Respiratory
  - Oxygen desaturation
  - Bronchospasm

Cardiovascular Complications

- It is important to take a history to note the presence and extent of any pre-existing cardiovascular disease (e.g. heart failure, ischaemic heart disease, and anaemia), including the use of any cardiovascular medications (e.g. negatively chronotropic drugs), to examine any pre-test cardiovascular investigations (e.g. electrocardiograms) and to measure the pre-procedure resting heart rate and blood pressure.
- It is important to take note of the pre-procedure resting blood pressure and any antihypertensive medication that may have been taken pre-test.

ECG Changes

- We can further divide ECG changes into rhythm changes and ST segment changes.
- Specific rhythm changes
  - Ectopics – often disappear with exercise. If ectopics change in morphology or begin to appear in clusters, consider ending the test early.

Table 4.1 Contraindications for CPET

Absolute	Relative
- Acute Myocardial Ischaemia/Infarction (3–5 days)	- Left main or three-vessel coronary artery disease (untreated)
- Unstable angina	- Asymptomatic severe aortic stenosis
- Unstable or symptomatic arrhythmia causing hypotension	- Severe arterial hypertension at rest (>200 mmHg systolic or 120 mmHg diastolic)
- Active endocarditis	- Tachyarrhythmia or bradyarrhythmia
- Acute myocarditis, pericarditis, pulmonary oedema	- Hypertrophic cardiomyopathy
- Syncope	- Significant pulmonary hypertension
- Severe, symptomatic aortic stenosis	- Thrombosis of the lower extremity (until treated for a minimum of 2 weeks)
- Uncontrolled or decompensated heart failure	- Within 2 weeks of acute symptomatic pulmonary embolus
- Suspected dissecting or leaking aortic aneurysm	- Abdominal aortic aneurysm >8.0 cm in diameter
- Uncontrolled asthma	- Electrolyte abnormality
- SpO_2 <85% on room air at rest	- Advanced or complicated pregnancy
- Acute significant non-cardiopulmonary disorder that may affect or be adversely affected by exercise	- Orthopaedic impairment
- Significant psychiatric/cognitive impairment limiting cooperation	- Potentially ICD that is not readily accessible/cannot be deactivated

Adapted with permission of the American Thoracic Society. Copyright © 2023 American Thoracic Society. All rights reserved. American Thoracic Society; American College of Chest Physicians. ATS/ACCP Statement on cardiopulmonary exercise testing. *Am J Respir Crit Care Med.* 15 Jan 2003;167(2):211–77. The *American Journal of Respiratory and Critical Care Medicine* is an official journal of the American Thoracic Society. Readers are encouraged to read the entire article for the correct context at https://doi.org/10.1164/rccm.167.2.211. The authors, editors, and the American Thoracic Society are not responsible for errors or omissions in adaptations.

- ○ Atrial Fibrillation – if AF develops during the test, it provides a potential explanation for exercise limitation.
- ○ Ventricular Tachycardia – if VT develops terminate the test, pulsed VT will require further investigation, and potentially intervention. Pulseless VT obviously requires immediate cardiopulmonary resuscitation.

- ST segment changes
  - ○ It is important to take note of the presence of any ST segment anomalies, with specific regard to how they may change during exercise.
  - ○ Myocardial ischaemia is present if ST segment depression of ≥ 2 mm develops; consider ending the test at that point if symptomatic or if >4 mm depression and asymptomatic.
  - ○ Additionally, consider ending a test if there is >1 mm ST elevation.

Blood Pressure Changes

- Normally, systolic blood pressure will progressively rise during exercise.
- Although movement artefact can affect BP readings, any drop of >20% from baseline should be reconfirmed.
- Beyond this, there are two potential complicating responses:
- Hypotension
  - ○ A fall in systolic blood pressure of >20% from baseline during exercise may indicate the presence of significant myocardial ischaemia or outflow tract obstruction (e.g. aortic stenosis).
  - ○ Additionally, hypotension may be associated with other symptoms, including pre-syncope, anginal pain, and so on.
- Hypertension
  - ○ It is possible for blood pressure to undergo an exaggerated response to exercise resulting in systolic and/or diastolic hypertension.
  - ○ It is important to monitor this throughout the test, being mindful of the onset of any symptoms of malignant hypertension (e.g. chest pain, shortness of breath, or dizziness) and the potential need for early termination of the test.
  - ○ An exaggerated hypertensive response to exercise is associated with increased cardiovascular risk.

Respiratory Complications

- It is important to take a history to note the presence and extent of any pre-existing lung disease, to perform pre-test spirometry and flow-volume loops, and to measure the pre-procedure resting SpO_2.

Oxygen Desaturation

- Falling SpO_2 value during exercise suggests significant pathology.
- If SpO_2 is normal at rest and proceeds to drop below 80% during exercise → stop the test.
- Beware if using a finger probe for pulse oximetry; in some patients on a cycle ergometer, gripping the handlebars tightly might result in a falsely low reading; in such cases, ask them to loosen their grip and assess whether desaturation is real or artefactual.
- We will discuss this in more detail in Part III.

Bronchospasm

- Bronchospasm may be exercise-induced (e.g. as in some forms of asthma).
- Most CPET systems will display flow-volume loops during the test. It is worth consulting these at regular intervals to see whether expiratory airflow limitation has developed – seen as a 'scalloping' of the expiratory limb of the loop (see the section Flow-Volume Loops in Chapter 5).
- A fall in FEV_1 of 20% or more during exercise suggests exercise-induced asthma.

Patient Information and Consent for CPET

As we have established, complications do occur during CPET; therefore, patients should be provided with information related to the investigation, including the conduct of the test, potential risks and benefits, identifying new undiagnosed conditions which may require further investigation, and so on. Additionally, in order to maintain standardisation of testing, information on how patients should prepare themselves for testing is important, including:

- Continuing regular medications
- Avoidance of caffeine, alcohol, or cigarettes
- Refraining from eating within the 2 hours prior to testing
- Drinking only water within the 2 hours prior to testing
- Avoiding strenuous exercise on the day of testing.

The manner in which this is conveyed to the patients, and how the process of informed consent is obtained varies between practitioners and institutions and may include patient information leaflets, telephonic consultations, and face-to-face consultations. Documentation of these processes is appropriate and some institutions ask for written, informed consent for cardiopulmonary exercise tests.

It is also important, for the purpose of meaningfully interpreting tests and creating a report, to record some baseline patient information. This should include the following:

- Basic demographics and anthropometric indicators – age, sex, height, weight, BMI, and so on.
- Reason for referral (e.g. assessment of peri-operative risk and proposed surgery).
- Medical history – paying particular attention to any disease processes that may impair exercise, not only cardiorespiratory disease but also musculoskeletal and potentially metabolic or endocrine disease.
- Drug history – identifying any drugs that may limit the physiological response to exercise (e.g. negative chronotropic drugs such as beta-blockers).
- Blood results – with particular attention to haemoglobin, as anaemia can limit performance.

Chapter 5

Spirometry and Flow-Volume Loops

Basics

Spirometry literally means 'measuring of breath', and as an investigation it reflects the lung's bellows function and can be used to determine the extent of respiratory disease.

To understand basic spirometry, we need to describe how the total space within the lungs is divided into volumes and capacities. A volume is a specific measurement of either inspired or expired gas (or in the case of tidal volume both), whereas a capacity is combination of two or more volumes. The differing lung volumes are shown in Figure 5.1 and the different lung volumes and capacity are described as follows:

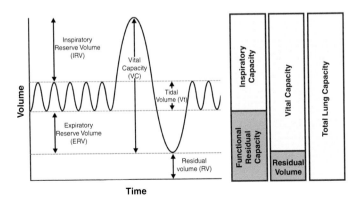

Figure 5.1 Different lung volumes and capacities

- **Tidal Volume (Vt)** – the volume of air moved in and out of respiratory tract during each ventilatory cycle (i.e. a single inhalation and exhalation).
  - This equates to approximately 7 ml/kg.
- **Inspiratory Reserve Volume (IRV)** – the additional volume that can be forcibly inhaled after a normal inspiration.
  - This equates to approximately 45 ml/kg.
- **Expiratory Reserve Volume (ERV)** – the additional volume that can be forcibly exhaled after a normal expiration.
  - This equates to approximately 15 ml/kg.
- **Vital Capacity (VC)** – the maximal volume that can be forcibly exhaled after a maximal inspiration.
  - This is the combination of the tidal volume and both the inspiratory and expiratory reserve volumes, that is, $VC = Vt + IRV + ERV$.
  - This equates to approximately 60–70 ml/kg.
- **Residual Volume (RV)** – the volume remaining in the lungs after maximal expiration.
  - $RV = FRC - ERV$
  - This equates to approximately 15 ml/kg.
  - This volume, and any capacity containing it, cannot be measured by spirometry alone. An alternative method is required; for example whole body plethysmography.
- **Function Residual Capacity (FRC)** – the volume remaining in the lungs at the end of normal expiration.
  - This is the combination of the residual volume and the expiratory reserve volume. That is, $FRC = RV + ERV$
  - This equates to approximately 30 ml/kg.
- **Total Lung Capacity (TLC)** – the volume in the lungs at the end of maximal inspiration.
  - This is the combination of all volumes/capacities.
  - $TLC = FRC + Vt + IRV$
  - Or alternatively, $TLC = VC + RV$
  - This equates to approximately 75–80 ml/kg.
- **Minute Volume** = the volume exhaled per minute.
  - Not shown in Figure 5.1.

How Is the Test Performed?

- A patient is asked to perform specific breathing manoeuvres into a spirometer – a device that measures the relative inspiratory and expiratory volumes.
- After maximal inspiration, a single forced complete expiration is recorded and two parameters are measured, and one parameter is calculated:
  - FEV_1 = volume after 1 second (usually around 80% of FVC)
  - FVC = the total volume forcibly expired
  - FEV_1/FVC (expressed as a percentage)
- Normal spirometry is shown in Figure 5.2.

What Does the Test Tell Us?

- Results are interpreted in the context of percentage of predicted normal values.
- (Test reading/predicted value) × 100 = % of predicted value.
- An abnormality is seen in the presence of any one of the following:
  - FEV_1 <80% predicted normal
  - FVC <80% predicted normal
  - FEV_1/FVC < 0.7.

Obstructive Disorder

- In simple terms, these are disorders limiting exhalation of air from the lungs.

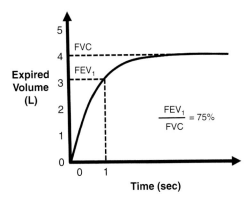

Figure 5.2 Normal spirometry

- Examples include COPD, asthma, and bronchiectasis.
- Such disorders are suggested by:
  - FEV1 <80%
  - FVC usually reduced (although to lesser degree than FEV_1)
  - FEV_1/FVC ratio <0.7.
- NICE COPD definitions of degree of airflow obstruction are as follows:
  - Mild airflow obstruction = FEV_1 between 50% and 80%
  - Moderate airflow obstruction = FEV_1 between 30% and 49%
  - Severe airflow obstruction = FEV_1 <30%.

Restrictive Disorder

- In simple terms, these are disorders in which the lungs are 'restricted' from expanding, and hence cannot be fully filled.
- Examples include interstitial lung disease, pulmonary fibrosis, obesity, neuromuscular diseases (e.g. amyotrophic lateral sclerosis), and disorders of the chest wall or spine (e.g. scoliosis).
- Such disorders are suggested by:
  - FEV_1 <80% (although to a lesser degree than FVC)
  - FVC <80%
  - FEV_1/FVC ratio >0.7.

Reversibility

- Certain disorders can exhibit a degree of reversibility (especially obstructive disorders, for example asthmatic bronchoconstriction).
- Spirometry is undertaken pre- and post-bronchodilator administration.
- Reversibility is defined as an FEV_1 increase of >200 ml or 15%.

Normal Spirometry

- Normal physiology allows for 75% of the FVC to be forcibly expired in 1 s (FEV_1).
- If we take an example FVC of 4 000 ml, under normal circumstances the FEV_1 should be approximately 3 000 ml (see Figure 5.2).

Obstructive Pattern

- In obstructive airway disease, there is limitation of the volume of gas that can be forcibly expired (shown in Figure 5.3).
- Therefore, the FVC and FEV_1 are both reduced.

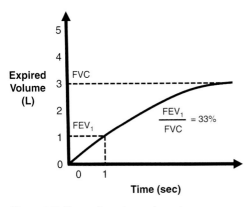

Figure 5.3 Obstructive pattern spirometry

- This results in a lower FEV1/FVC ratio (the ratio is 33% in the example shown in Figure 5.3).

Restrictive Pattern

- In restrictive lung disease, there is limitation of the volume of gas that can be held in the lungs; hence, overall FVC is reduced, whilst early expiration is not usually affected (and thus FEV_1 usually remains normal or near normal).
- This results in an FEV_1/FVC ratio that is normal or high (the ratio is 85% in the example shown in Figure 5.4).

Flow-Volume Loops

- These are plots of flow (during both inspiration and expiration) against volume.
- These loops can be plotted during both spontaneous and mechanical ventilation (although there are slight variations to the plots themselves).
- Tests begin with a forced exhalation from vital capacity. The loop in a spontaneously ventilating patient is drawn clockwise from total lung capacity (TLC) to residual volume (RV) and back to TLC again (the normal loop is shown in Figure 5.5).
- Flow rates are the maximum attainable at each lung volume.
- Expiration is represented by the positive deflection. Initially the flow rate is rapid, and after peaking, it steadily decreases as expiration continues. This part of the loop is often a relatively straight line, but may show slight concavity.

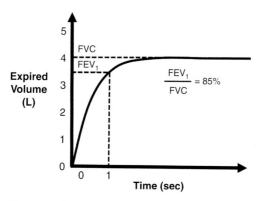

Figure 5.4 Restrictive pattern spirometry

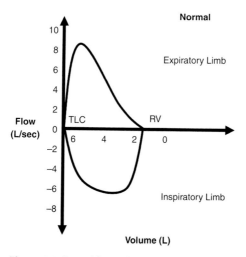

Figure 5.5 Normal flow-volume loop

- Inspiration is represented by the negative deflection. This part of the loop is often squarer in shape. The maximum flow is usually in the range of 4–6L/s.
- The appearance of the flow-volume loops changes in different disease processes.

Obstructive Airways Disease

- Obstructive airways disease reduces peak expiratory flow rate (PEFR) and increases RV (via gas trapping), as shown in Figure 5.6.
- TLC may also be higher.
- Flow rates fall during expiration.
- The expiratory limb exhibits increased concavity from airway obstruction.
- The inspiratory limb is less affected, with potentially slightly lower flow rates.

Restrictive Airways Disease

- Restrictive disease reduces TLC (curve shifts to the right), but preserves RV, as shown in Figure 5.7.
- PEFR is generally reduced.

Variable Extrathoracic Obstruction

- Usually allows expiratory flow as positive pressure during expiration splints airways open, as shown in Figure 5.8.
- Negative pressure on inspiration worsens obstruction/collapse.

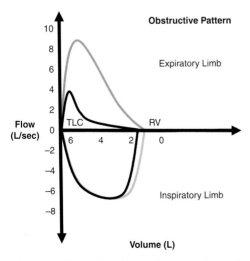

Figure 5.6 Flow-volume loop in obstructive airways disease

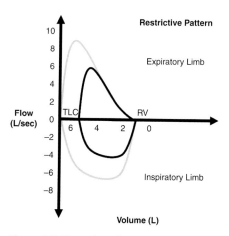

Figure 5.7 Flow-volume loop in restrictive airways disease

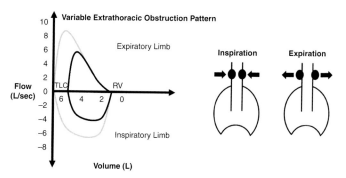

Figure 5.8 Flow-volume loop in variable extrathoracic obstruction and effect of respiratory phase on obstruction

Variable Intrathoracic Obstruction

- Usually allows inspiration as negative intrathoracic pressure during inspiration splints airways open, as shown in Figure 5.9.
- Positive pressure on expiration worsens obstruction/collapse.

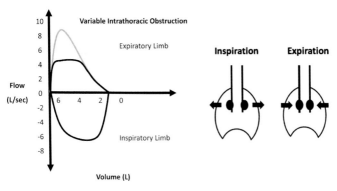

Figure 5.9 Flow-volume loop in variable intrathoracic obstruction and effect of respiratory phase on obstruction

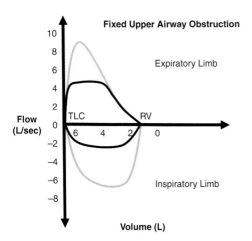

Figure 5.10 Flow-volume loop in fixed airways obstruction

Fixed Airway Obstruction

- A fixed orifice results in turbulent flow. Inspiratory and expiratory flow rates depend on the orifice diameter, but BOTH are reduced, as shown in Figure 5.10.
- For example, tracheal stenosis.

Chapter 6

Ergometers and Work Rate Increment, Equipment, Staff, and Preparation

Cardiopulmonary exercise testing is usually performed using either a treadmill or a cycle ergometer; each has their benefits and limitations (outlined in Table 6.1). Most institutions use a cycle ergometer for CPET – although semi-recumbent ergometers can also be used and it is also possible to use a hand crank for patients with limited leg mobility. It is worth noting that CPET values reported in research papers in peri-operative medicines tend to have been derived from cycle ergometers.

Table 6.1 The major differences between treadmill and cycle ergometers

	Treadmill	**Cycle**
Max VO_2	Higher (More muscle groups used)	Lower
Work rate measurement	No	Yes
Blood gas collection	More difficult	Easier
Potential for artefact	More	Less
Safety	Possibly less safe	Possibly safer
Weight bearing	More	Less
Degree of leg muscle training	More	Less
More appropriate for	Active normal subjects	Wider array of patients

Calculating Work Rate Increment

The rate of increment in work rate is predetermined using an estimate of expected work capacity with the following equations:

- Work rate increment $(W/min) = (Peak\ VO_2 - VO_2\ unloaded)/100$
- VO_2 unloaded$(ml/min) = 150 + [6 \times weight(kg)]$
- Peak $VO_2(ml/min)$men $=$ height$(cm) -$ age$(years) \times 20$
- Peak $VO_2(ml/min)$women $=$ height$(cm) -$ age$(years) \times 14$

Equipment, Staff, and Preparation
Equipment and Calibration

- Test equipment includes the following:
  - Electronically braked cycle ergometer
  - 12 lead ECG – to allow for measurement of rate, rhythm, and QRS complex/ST segment changes (lead set-up shown in Figure 6.1)
  - Pulse oximetry
  - Blood pressure cuff
  - Metabolic cart with oxygen and carbon dioxide analysers (response time of 90 ms or less, to allow breath-by-breath analysis).
- Resuscitation equipment should be immediately available and include the following:
  - Defibrillator and resuscitation equipment
  - Oxygen
  - Emergency drugs.
- Calibration of equipment is essential to have accurate data upon which clinical decisions may be made.
- Calibration should be made before EACH test (including flowmeters and gas analysers) or as recommended by the system manufacturer.
- Adjustments should be possible for variations in barometric pressure, humidity, and temperature.
- Flowmeters are calibrated using a gas syringe of known volume over a variety of flow rates.
- Gas analysers are tested by two-point calibration using inhaled gas (room air) and a specially formulated standard exhaled air cylinder.

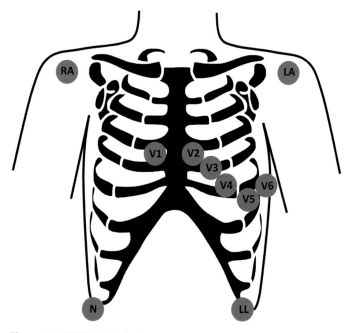

Figure 6.1 12 ECG electrode placement

Staff and Supervision

The staff member performing the test should be trained in basic life support, ECG interpretation, CPET test protocols, including the ability to interpret the test and knowledge of the reasons to terminate a test. If the test reporter is not administering the test, any additional information from direct observation during testing should be communicated to the reporter.

A doctor should be immediately available in the event of a complication during the test, or present during a high-risk test where a patient has a relative contraindication, for safety purposes.

Testing in the Context of the Covid-19 Pandemic and Other Infectious Respiratory Diseases

The Covid-19 pandemic in 2019 resulted in a worldwide public health emergency. The SARS-CoV-2 virus was a novel, highly contagious virus – initially defined as an acute respiratory disease. Subsequent experience and observation has shown it to be a multi-system disease with potentially long-lasting effects. The need to maintain surgical services for high-risk patients during the pandemic resulted in changes in the provision of CPET. As the virus became endemic, and with the potential for future outbreaks of other novel viruses, it is important to have standard operating procedures in place to mitigate the impact of viruses in the community and limit disruption to CPET services.

Indications
- The indications for CPET remain unchanged, and have potentially been expanded to include investigation and assessment of the long Covid-19 syndrome, the effects of rehabilitation programmes related to the disease, and so on.

Contraindications
- Active Covid-19 infection is a contraindication to CPET, additionally patients with Covid-19 symptoms or a new pyrexia should be postponed.

Screening
- All patients should be screened, in some form, for Covid-19 prior to testing.
- Patients with resolved infection (but persistently positive tests) can be considered on a case-by-case basis depending on clinical need, and be scheduled for testing when non-infectious.

Precautions
- CPET itself is an aerosol-generating procedure, and as such can potentially result in infection of CPET personnel. As such safety precautions are necessary to limit transmission.
- CPET should be undertaken in a closed room with the minimum number of staff possible.
- The ventilation of the room where CPET is undertaken should be assessed.
- Equipment should be inspected for cleanliness and any potential areas of damage which could become contaminated.
- Staff should don appropriate personal protective equipment (PPE) as outlined by the relevant public health body in their

country of practice – this usually consists of N-95 mask, gloves, gown, and face shield or eye protection.

- Patients should remain masked until ready for CPET.
- Following completion of CPET, the testing room and equipment should be decontaminated.
  - Single-use equipment should be discarded.
  - Reusable equipment (e.g. facemasks and ventilation tubes) should be cleaned appropriately; this may include washing with soap or detergent and warm water, the use of enzymatic cleaning solutions, and so on.
- The air change rate for the testing room should be used to calculate the duration between tests, or utilisation of air purifiers with high-grade HEPA filters and UV light, which can reduce the time to 5 minutes.
- In the absence of such measures, the testing room should be 'aired out' following cleaning for a defined time period as specified by relevant bodies – different organisations may have different recommendations for duration between tests (e.g. the European Respiratory Society suggests 30–60 minutes).

Testing in the context of 'post-Covid-19 condition' or 'long Covid-19'

- This is an evolving field of study and there are four main areas that need to be cautiously and diligently explored before patients engage in rehabilitation programmes or undergo CPET.

  1. Post-exertional symptom exacerbation (PESE)

     - Here, symptoms (cardiac, respiratory, neurological, and musculoskeletal) are exacerbated after exertion. The exacerbation may be out-of-proportion to the effort made, but can be disabling and may present immediately or be delayed (occurring 24–72 hours later). CPET can be a trigger, and a full history of any PESE needs to be ascertained.

  2. Impairment of cardiac function

     - Patients with Covid-19 are at increased risk of cardiovascular disease. If chest pain is present and has hitherto not been investigated, there is a small but significant risk of cardiac death, such that some organisations (e.g. the Society for Occupational Medicine) recommend that exertion be contraindicated.

3. Exertional oxygen desaturation

   - It has been suggested that in patients with long Covid-19, a fall in oxygen saturations of ≤3% is abnormal and significant, requiring investigation. Other aspects of respiratory function should be examined, including the potential for hyperventilation or abnormal breathing patterns. Referral for lung function tests, diffusing capacity, and specialist respiratory physiotherapy should be considered.

4. Dysautonomia

   - Patients with long Covid-19 may suffer with autonomic dysfunction and orthostatic intolerances, for example postural orthostatic tachycardia syndrome. The symptoms of such conditions need to be differentiated from underlying cardiac or respiratory disease. The presence of dysautonomia may require adaptation to the conduct of CPET, for example the use of a supine ergometer and the use of compression garments.

Patient Preparation and Test Set-Up

Prior to performing the test, a detailed history and basic clinical examination are required.

- It is worth reviewing any available investigations, for example CXR, ECG, and blood tests (particularly haemoglobin level).
- An explanation of the overall conduct of the test and potential complications should be undertaken. In some centres, this will involve written informed consent.
- Ideally, perform spirometry and flow-volume loops before testing.
- ECG leads may be applied before mounting the bike, or whilst the patient is on the bike (depending on preference). Shaving or skin cleaning may be required to achieve the optimum contact.
- Instructions for performance of the test and the means to communicate during the test are given (and the patient is coached on using the mouthpiece, if applicable).

  ○ The patient is instructed that there are four basic phases to the test akin to riding a bicycle: baseline (sat stationary), unloaded (cycling downhill), loaded (cycling uphill), and recovery (stopping).

- The patient should be encouraged to 'try their best' and be reassured that everyone reaches a point at which they cannot cycle any further and that this is normal.
- Explain the importance of remaining seated, maintaining a steady pedal cadence, and that they may be asked to 'speed up' or 'slow down'. The patient is shown their leg speed (rpm) and told to aim to maintain at approximately 60 rpm for the duration of the test. This is important, as the wattage is calculated by the cycle ergometer depending on cadence and resistance – it can accommodate for variation in cadence (approximately 40–90 revolutions per minute) but adaptation takes time. Hence a steady pace is preferable.
- Instruct the patient not to speak during the test, as this may interfere with gas analysis.
- Explain that if the patient experiences any dizziness or faintness whilst exercising, they should *stop* pedalling.
- Any other symptoms should be reported by hand signals where possible, at which point monitoring can be reviewed.
- Explain the process of stopping the test, including the need to gradually 'warm down' from peak exercise, rather than stopping abruptly (which can precipitate hypotension).

7

Workload, Breath-by-Breath Analysis and Test Phases, and Stopping a Cardiopulmonary Exercise Test

Workload

- The resistance applied to the pedals of the cycle ergometer can be increased in two ways (shown in Figure 7.1):
  - Incremental – there is a step-wise gradual increase in resistance at specified time intervals.
  - Ramp – there is a gradual constant increase in resistance with time.
- A continuous ramp is the gold standard.
- The gradient is pre-determined using an estimate of expected work capacity.
- The duration of the test is variable (often between 6 minutes and 10 minutes of loaded cycling). Too short a test (e.g. with sprinting) may result in early anaerobic activity. Too long a test and the patient may become bored and terminate early (before reaching peak activity).

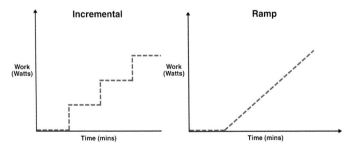

Figure 7.1 Incremental versus ramp workload

Breath-by-Breath Display

- Gas analysers allow for the composition of exhaled gas to be examined on a breath-by-breath basis.
- These measurements are usually then averaged over a few breaths to allow for a more easily interpretable/smoother graphical display.

Test Phases

- The test consists of four phases: rest, unloaded activity, loaded activity, and recovery.
- The recommended times allotted to these phases varies between clinical organisations.
- To help a patient conceptualise what the test involves, it can be helpful to ask them to imagine themselves on a bicycle at the top of a hill, see Figure 7.2.

1. Rest (2–3 minutes)
   - Baseline measurements taken with the patient sitting still on the ergometer.
   - Allows for stabilisation in breathing pattern changes whilst fitting the mask.

2. Unloaded activity (2–3 minutes)
   - During unloaded activity, they begin to cycle 'downhill' with no resistance.
   - Allows for stabilisation of breathing pattern with additional muscular work.

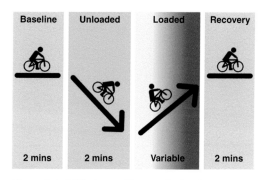

Figure 7.2 CPET phases with example durations

3. Loaded activity/ramping (variable, usually 6–12 minutes)
   - During loaded cycling, resistance is gradually introduced and they begin to cycle 'uphill', where the steepness of the hill may seem to gradually increase, as work rate gradually increases with time.

4. Recovery (2 minutes onwards)
   - There will come a point when they will no longer be able to maintain an adequate pedal cadence, at which point workload is removed.
   - It is important that the patient continues pedalling to warm down (albeit with decreasing speed) to prevent any sudden cardiovascular changes that may occur with an abrupt stop.
   - Changes in workload related to different test phases are shown in Figure 7.3.

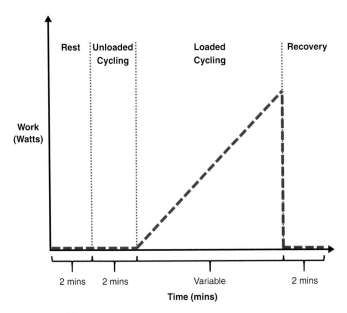

Figure 7.3 How workload varies with time and test phase

Stopping a Cardiopulmonary Exercise Test

Either the patient or the responsible clinician can stop a cardiopulmonary exercise test. In either case, whether a test has been taken to completion or has required early termination, it is important to understand and document the reasons.

In general, there are three main symptoms that will cause a patient to stop exercising during a test:

- Fatigue
  - The onset of fatigue is seen when the force output of muscles begins to diminish for a given stimulus.
  - The exact mechanism is unknown.

- Dyspnoea
  - Under normal circumstances, dyspnoea itself is not usually the cause of exercise cessation. It is, however, a common exercise-induced symptom.
  - There are several different pathophysiological states that often occur in conjunction to cause dyspnoea.
  - This is covered in more detail later in Part IV.

- Pain
  - Pain can include musculoskeletal or can be related to vascular supply, for example angina or claudication.

Patient Effort

- Adequate motivation during the test is key to attaining a patient's maximal effort, and in turn determining the true extent of any exercise limitation.
- To this end, a submaximal effort can cast doubt on any results and may interfere with CPET interpretation.
- There are no agreed standards for the criteria that constitute a maximal effort, although a maximal effort is likely if one or more of the following are present:
  - RER >1.15
  - Achieved predicted peak work rate
  - Achieved predicted peak VO_2
  - Achieved predicted peak heart rate.

Why Might Exercise Be Limited?

- There are several different ways in which the performance of exercise might be limited. We can broadly classify these into four categories:
- Cardiovascular causes
  - Reduced stroke volume
  - Abnormal heart rate response
  - Circulatory and blood abnormality
- Pulmonary causes
  - Impaired gas exchange or ventilation
  - Respiratory muscle dysfunction
- Peripheral causes
  - Inactivity, atrophy, or deconditioning
  - Neuromuscular dysfunction
  - Reduced oxidative capacity of skeletal muscle
  - Malnutrition
- Other causes
  - Perceptual
  - Motivational
  - Environmental.

When Might a Test End Early?

In general, the majority of tests end early due to cardiac limitation rather than ventilatory limitation.

- Cardiac limitation
  - Stopping secondary to leg fatigue
  - Pump limitation (e.g. demonstrated by an O_2 pulse plateau).
- Ventilatory limitation
  - Stopping secondary to dyspnoea
  - Ventilatory inefficiency (e.g. demonstrated by failure of $PETCO_2$ to fall after peaking near AT/peak exercise).

When to Terminate a Test Early?

If a patient terminates a test early, it is usually due to symptoms (with or without poor motivation). There are, however, several reasons why the responsible clinician may need to prematurely stop a test, which are primarily concerned with patient safety and the presence of test complications, but may also include futility (e.g. patient is unable to maintain an adequate rpm). The criteria for prematurely stopping a test are outlined next.

Patient Stopping Criteria

- Patient stops due to fatigue, pain, or light headedness.
  - For fatigue or pain, it may be possible to encourage a patient to continue for a bit longer (e.g. a further 30 s).
- Patient fails to maintain an rpm of >40 for more than 1 minute and does not respond to encouragement.

Test Complication Criteria

- ECG related
  - Cardiac ischaemia – chest pain or ECG changes (>2 mm symptomatic ST depression, >4 mm asymptomatic ST depression, or >1 mm ST elevation)
  - Significant arrhythmia resulting in symptoms or haemodynamic compromise (may include complex ectopy/second- or third-degree heart block).
- Blood pressure related
  - Fall in systolic BP >20 mmHg from highest value during test
  - Hypertension >250 mmHg systolic or >120 mmHg diastolic
  - Sudden pallor.
- Respiratory
  - Severe desaturation <80%
  - Signs and/or symptoms of hypoxaemia
  - Signs of respiratory failure.
- Conscious state or level
  - Change in conscious level (including confusion)
  - Dizziness or faintness.

Chapter

8

Different Plots and CPET Interpretation

The variables that a cardiopulmonary exercise test aims to measure can be presented in a number of different ways. The standard method of presenting these data is as a 9-panel plot. Different 9-panel plots are available; which arrange individual plots in different orientations. The three most commonly used plots are the following:

- Traditional Wasserman 9-panel plot
- New Wasserman UCLA 9-panel plot
- Whipp (European Respiratory Society) plot

Traditional Wasserman 9-Panel Plot

The x-axis can either use work rate or time as the variable. In either instance, the curves are the same. An example of the original Wasserman Harbour UCLA 9-panel plot is shown in Figure 8.1.

- Panel 1 – VE versus work rate (or time)
- Panel 2 – HR and VO_2/HR versus work rate (or time)
- Panel 3 – VO_2 and VCO_2 versus work rate (or time)
- Panel 4 – VE versus VCO_2
- Panel 5 – VCO_2 and HR versus VO_2
- Panel 6 – VEVEO$_2$ and VEVCO$_2$ versus work rate (or time)
- Panel 7 – Vt versus VE
- Panel 8 – RER versus work rate (or time)
- Panel 9 – PETO$_2$ and PETCO$_2$ versus work rate (or time)

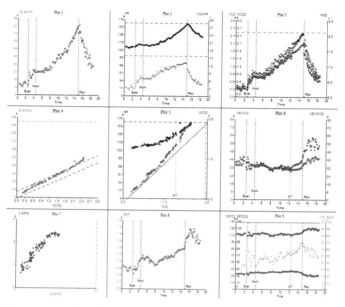

Figure 8.1 Traditional Wasserman 9-panel plot

Every 9-panel plot has various graphs or combinations of graphs that can be used to understand the physiology and pathophysiology that underpins a cardiopulmonary exercise test. Figure 8.2 illustrates which plots can be used to interpret different parameters.

New Wasserman UCLA 9-Panel Plot

Like in the original plot, the x-axis can again either use work rate or time as the variable, with the resultant curves being the same. An example of the New Wasserman UCLA 9-panel plot is shown in Figure 8.3, and how plots can be interpreted is shown in Figure 8.4.

- Panel 1 – VO$_2$ and VCO$_2$ versus work rate (or time)
- Panel 2 – HR and VO$_2$/HR (oxygen pulse) versus work rate (or time)

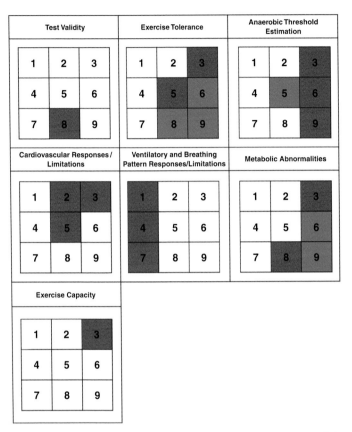

Figure 8.2 Different plot combinations in the Traditional Wasserman 9-panel plot and the parameters they measure

- Panel 3 – VCO_2 and HR versus VO_2
- Panel 4 – $VEVCO_2$ and $VEVO_2$ versus time
- Panel 5 – VE versus time
- Panel 6 – VE versus VCO_2
- Panel 7 – $PETO_2$ and $PETCO_2$ versus time
- Panel 8 – RER versus time
- Panel 9 – Vt versus VE

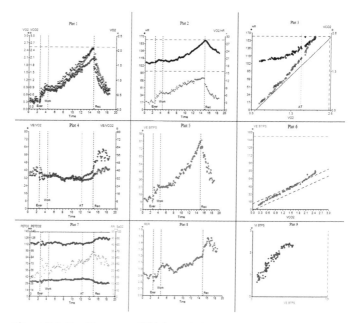

Figure 8.3 New Wasserman UCLA 9-panel plot

The Whipp (European Respiratory Society) 9-Panel Plot

- The benefit of this approach is that the three panels arranged vertically on the left-hand column of the plot (panels 1, 4, and 7) all deal with anaerobic threshold aiding in AT estimation.
- This plot has been adopted as the European Respiratory Society format.
- The ninth panel (lower right-hand corner) is non-assigned, that is it can be chosen by the practitioner.
- An example of the Whipp 9-panel plot is shown in Figure 8.5, and how plots can be interpreted is shown in Figure 8.6.
  - Panel 1 – VCO_2 versus VO_2
  - Panel 2 – VO_2 versus work rate

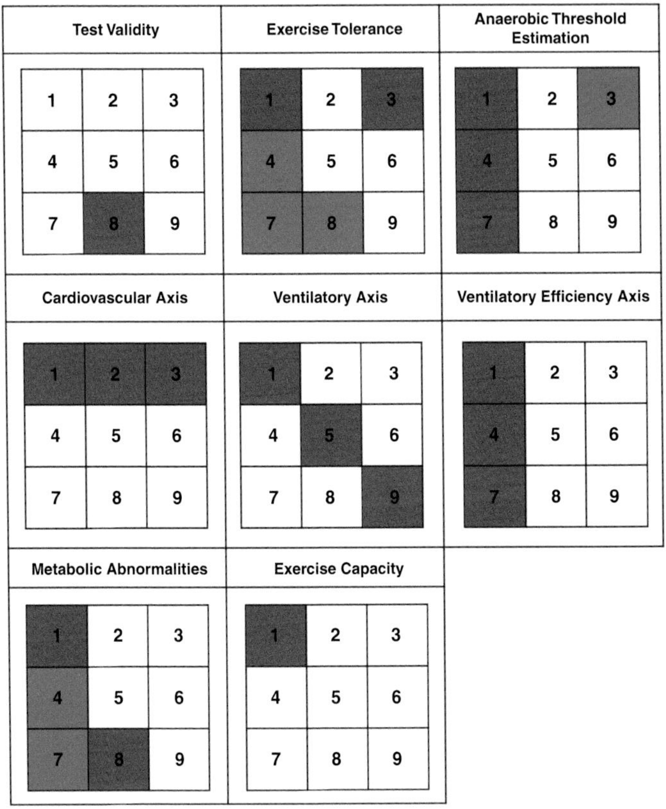

Figure 8.4 Different plot combinations in the new Wasserman UCLA 9-panel plot and the parameters they measure

- Panel 3 – HR and VO_2/HR (oxygen pulse) versus VO_2
- Panel 4 – $VEVCO_2$ and $VEVO_2$ versus VO_2
- Panel 5 – VE versus VCO_2
- Panel 6 – Vt versus VE
- Panel 7 – $PETO_2$ and $PETCO_2$ versus VO_2
- Panel 8 – RER versus work rate (or time)
- Panel 9 – VE versus work rate (or time)

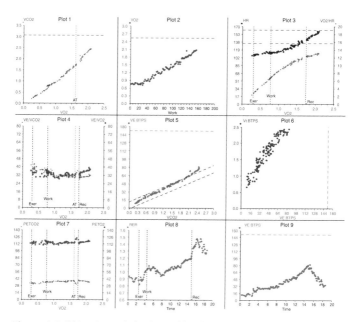

Figure 8.5 Whipp 9-panel plot (as used by the European Respiratory Society)

CPET Interpretation

Whilst several different plots can be used, and panels may be arranged in different orders, for the most part the same overall information is presented. Different panels may have additional notations, such as the following:

- Horizontal lines to show predicted maximums (e.g. heart rate) or lung volumes (e.g. IC and VC). These may be extended to show ranges (e.g. 80–100% of predicted).
- Vertical lines can show several different variables, such as the start of loaded work/recovery, AT, or lung volumes (e.g. MVV).

We will now approach the plots in an order that aims to answer the major questions of interest in cardiopulmonary exercise testing, explaining the underlying principles, their appearance

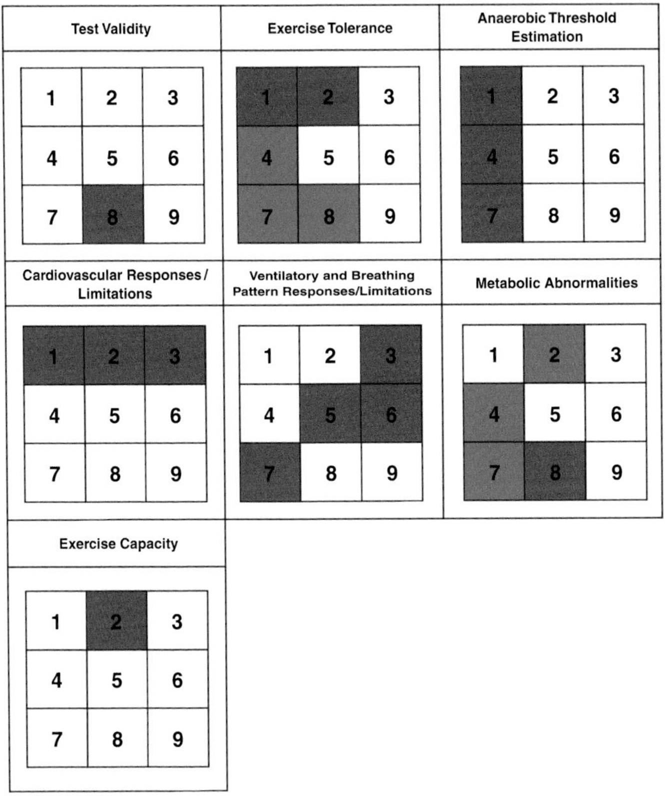

Figure 8.6 Different plot combinations in the Whipp 9-panel plot and the parameters they measure

under normal conditions, and how the plot can vary in different situations. This approach is outlined in Table 8.1, suggested normal values are shown in Tables 8.2 and 8.3, and the integration of the approach with normal values can be found in Figure 8.7.

Interpreting a Cardiopulmonary Exercise Test

Table 8.1 An approach to CPET interpretation

Question	Plot or parameter to review (target value)
Was the patient's effort maximal?	<ul><li>RER >1.15</li><li>Maximal work rate achieved (>80% predicted)</li><li>Maximal heart rate (>85% predicted)</li><li>Clear RCP</li><li>Peak VO_2 achieved (>80% predicted)</li></ul>
Is the patient's exercise capacity normal?	<ul><li>Peak VO_2 (>80% predicted)</li><li>Peak work rate (>80% predicted)</li><li>VO2 versus work rate slope (9–12 and linear)</li><li>OUES</li></ul>
When does anaerobic metabolism begin?	<ul><li>Anaerobic threshold plots</li><li>VCO_2 /VO_2 (AT >40% predicted peak VO_2)</li><li>$VEVO_2$ and $VEVCO_2$ versus VO_2</li><li>$PETO_2$ and $PETCO_2$ versus VO_2</li></ul>
Is circulation or oxygen transport normal?	<ul><li>VO2 versus work rate (9–12 and linear)</li><li>VO_2 versus HR (oxygen pulse >80% predicted)</li><li>Maximal heart rate (>85% predicted)</li><li>Heart rate reserve (<20%)</li><li>Heart rate recovery (>10% at 1minute)</li><li>ECG</li></ul>
Is ventilation, V/Q matching and gas exchange normal?	<ul><li>$VEVCO_2$ and $VEVO_2$ versus time ($VEVCO_2$ at AT <32)</li><li>VE/VCO_2 slope (<32)</li><li>Vt/VE</li><li>$PETO_2$ and $PETCO_2$ versus time</li><li>Breathing reserve (>30% or 15 litres)</li><li>SpO_2 (>95% at rest with minimal change)</li></ul>
Is the mechanism of exercise limitation visible and does it make sense with the clinical picture?	<ul><li>Whole 9-panel plot</li><li>Clinical history</li><li>Other investigations</li></ul>

Table 8.2 Suggested normal values (Adapted with permission from the Peri-operative Exercise Testing and Training Society)

Variable	Formula/derivation	Criteria for normality/impairment
Peak VO₂	Based on gender, age, height. Predicted peak VO_2: ♂ = (height − age) × 21 ♀ = (height − age) × 14 Normal >80% predicted >20 ml/kg/min Mild 70–80% 16–20 ml/kg/min	Moderate 50–69% 10–15 ml/kg/min Severe <50% <10 ml/kg/min
Resting VO₂	150 + (6 × weight in kg)	150 + (6 × weight in kg) = 250 to 300
VO₂/WR slope	9–12 ml/min/watt and linear (<9 or a change in gradient is abnormal)	
Anaerobic threshold	>40% predicted VO_2 max; Wide range of normal (40–80%) Normal >14 Mild 10–14	Moderate 8–10 Severe <8
Peak heart rate	220 − age	>85% predicted +/− 15 bpm
Heart rate reserve (HRR)	HRR <15 beats/min or <20% of peak heart rate	
Heart rate recovery	>10% at 1 minute in recovery phase	
O₂ pulse (VO₂/HR)	Predicted VO_2max / predicted max HR	>80% predicted ♂ = 15–20 ml/beat ♀ = 10–15 ml/beat

Table 8.2 (cont.)

Variable	Formula/derivation	Criteria for normality/impairment
Breathing reserve (BR)	$BR\ (\%) = \dfrac{100(MVV - VEmax)}{MVV}$ Or $BR = MVV - VEMax$	25–30% of MVV MVV estimated from FEV1 × 40 >30% or 15 L is normal
Minute ventilation (VE)	70–80% of MVV at peak exercise	
Respiratory frequency	<60 breaths/min	
Minimum VEVCO$_2$ (at AT)	23–34 – increases with age. >34 is abnormal	
VEVCO$_2$ slope	25 in young, increasing with age to a normal maximum of 32 >34 is abnormal, associated with increased risk, >42 is very high risk	
VEVO$_2$	20–30	
PETCO$_2$	35–42 mmHg (should fall after anaerobic threshold)	
PETO$_2$	90–110 mmHg (should rise after anaerobic threshold)	
SaO$_2$	>95% (should remain constant with exercise)	
Respiratory exchange ratio (RER)	Rest – 0.7–1.0 (<0.7 ?calibration error, >1.0 ?hyperventilation) Peak Exercise – >1.15	

Table 8.3 Suggested normal values and estimated risk threshold in Peri-operative Practice

POETTS&

POETTS&

Normal Values and Estimated Risk Thresholds

Remember Risk Thresholds are estimates & will vary for different procedures and will evolve as perioperative care evolves eg change in surgical technique and so are NOT fixed

Variable and Units	Normal Value							Abnormal/Associated with risk (approximates for risk)
VO_2-peak (ml/kg/min) Cycle ergometry Nb treadmill approx. 10% higher than cycle ergometer	Age	20-29 yrs	30-39 yrs	40-49 yrs	50-59 yrs	60-69 yrs	>70 yrs	• < 15ml/kg/min associated with increased perioperative risk • < 10 ml/kg/min very high risk
	M	42.0	30.8	28.0	26.1	22.9	21	
	F	30.8	22.2	20.1	18	16.6	16	
AT (ml/kg/min)	• 15-25ml/kg/min • Patients normal range 40-60% • Normal range 40-80% of VO_2peak							• < 9-10 associated with increased perioperative risk
VO_2/WR (ml/min/watt)	• 10 ml/min/watt • Normal range 9-12							• <9 abnormal (only linear portion of slope) • ↓ Gradient suggests impaired dynamic ventricular function • Abrupt change in gdnt suggests sudden impaired CO – ischaemia/arrhythmia/aortic stenosis/HOCUM
Peak HR (bpm)	• 220-age • Normal is 90% of predicted +/- 15bpm							• Note standard deviation 20-30
Peak Oxygen Pulse (ml/bt)	• VO_2= (SVxHR)(AV O_2 extraction ratio) • O_2 pulse = VO_2/HR= SV(O_2extraction ratio) • Normal > 80% of predicted approx: ○ Males: 15-20 ○ Females: 10-15							• Peak O_2 pulse reduced in heart failure and deconditioning • < 80% predicted value is abnormal • Early flattening of O_2 Pulse with ↑ HR suggests acute SV limitation – ischaemia, arrhythmia, heart failure
Breathing Reserve (ml/L or % of MVV)	• 25-30% of MVV • estimate MVV from FEV1X40							• < 15% of MVV = ventilatory limitation – limiting resp disease
VE/VCO_2 at AT or Minimum VE/VCO_2	• 23-34 • Increases with age to max 32							• > 34 abnormal & associated with ↑ perioperative risk (heart failure/respiratory disease)
VE/VCO_2 slope	• 25 in young • Increases with age to max 32 • Gradient – exc kinetic phase & above RCP							• > 35 associated with V/Q mismatch – heart failure, pulmonary hypertension, respiratory disease • ↑perioperative risk in thoracics > 35
Resp Rate (bpm)	• 8-12 rest							
Rest ETO$_2$ (mmHg)	• 90-110 mmHg, Increases above AT							• Low resting values in acute hyperventilation, heart failure and LV
Rest ETCO$_2$ (mmHg)	• 35-42 mmHg, Decreases above AT							
Rest RER	• 0.7-1.0							• < 0.7 ? calibration. > 1.0 ? hyperventilation
Peak RER	• > 1.15							• > 1.15 suggests physiologically maximal effort

(Reproduced with permission from the Peri-operative Exercise Testing and Training Society)

Interpreting a Cardiopulmonary Exercise Test

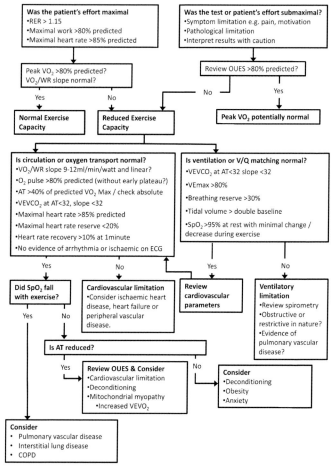

Figure 8.7 Example of diagnostic algorithm based on the approach to CPET interpretation in Table 8.1

RER versus Time (or Work Rate) Plot

- The respiratory exchange ratio (RER) is the ratio of carbon dioxide output (VCO_2) to oxygen uptake (VO_2) measured in expired gas.
  - $RER = VCO_2/VO_2$.
- Under steady state conditions, it is the same as the respiratory quotient (RQ), which is the ratio of CO_2 production to O_2 uptake, measured at the cellular or tissue level.
- In practice, the RER or RQ can be used to indicate what fuel source (carbohydrate or fat) is being utilised for metabolic processes (although accuracy is lost as exercise intensity increases due to several factors, for example the accumulation of lactate and the effect of bicarbonate buffering).
  - <0.8 implies fat is the main fuel source
  - 0.8–1.0 implies a mixture of carbohydrate and fat
  - >1.0 implies carbohydrate is the main fuel source
- The plot dealing with RER is panel 8 in all plots.
- In general, patient effort is said to be good if the peak exercise RER is >1.15.

Normal Responses

- VCO_2 at rest is slightly less than VO_2.
- Hence, starting RER is <1.0, with a normal range of 0.7–1.0 (with an average of 0.8).
- This is due to:
  a. Cells producing less CO_2 than they consume O_2
  b. Dissolving of CO_2 in bodily H_2O, contributing to the HCO_3^- buffering pool.

Interpreting a Cardiopulmonary Exercise Test

- At the start of exercise there is usually a slight dip in RER followed by an increase to 1.0 as muscular activity and cellular respiration increases (with rises in both VO_2 and VCO_2 – as shown in Figure 9.1).

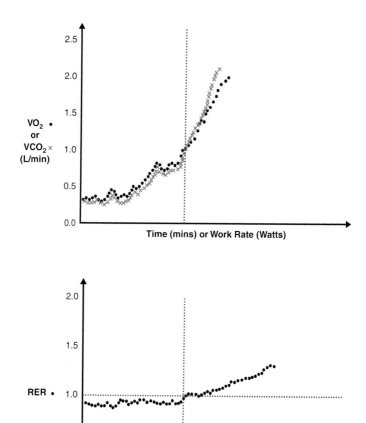

Figure 9.1 VO_2 and VCO_2 versus time and RER versus time curves

- The rise in RER becomes increasingly steep as HCO_3^- buffers lactic acid.
- The steepness depends on the rate of lactate production and the ability of the respiratory system to compensate for increasing acidosis.
- At the anaerobic threshold (AT) – the intersection where VCO_2 and VO_2 are equal (and beyond which VCO_2 rises disproportionately to VO_2), the RER must be less than or equal to 1.0.
- Beyond the anaerobic threshold, RER must be >1.0 since CO_2 production increases to buffer the acidaemia caused by an increase in lactic acid (whilst VO_2 cannot increase).
- In the recovery phase, normally RER increases further, before eventually decreasing. This is because, on cessation of exercise, CO_2 elimination is still high, whilst the oxygen debt is rapidly repaid and VO_2 falls.

Variations or Abnormal Responses
Falling RER at the Onset of Recovery

- A falling RER at cessation of exercise implies that there is either a fall in CO_2 elimination or a sustained/high level of O_2 consumption – both can be seen in cardiovascular limitation, and warrant investigation and corroboration with other plots.

Failure or Inability to Produce an Exercise Lactic Acidosis

- In this scenario, the RER cannot rise above 1.0.

Hyperventilation

- Leads to increased CO_2 washout without an increase in O_2 uptake – hence RER >1.0 before beginning exercise. Check against $PETCO_2$, which will show a decreasing $PETCO_2$ (shown in Figure 9.2).
- Lung disease can result in increased dead space. In this scenario, patients may hyperventilate to clear CO_2, the result of which is that RER can appear to be 'normal'.

Interpreting a Cardiopulmonary Exercise Test

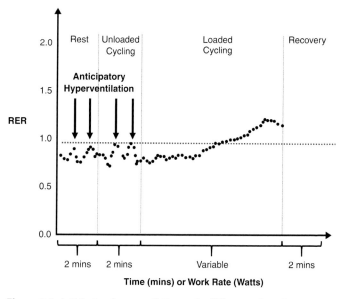

Figure 9.2 Anticipatory hyperventilation on the RER versus time plot

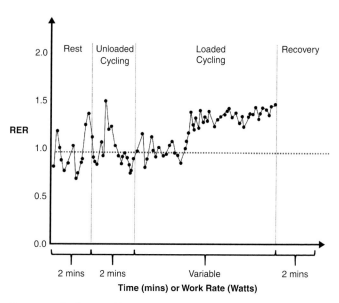

Figure 9.3 Dysfunctional breathing on the RER versus time plot

Dysfunctional or Oscillatory Breathing

- Pattern of abnormal ventilation unrelated to respiratory pathology.
- There is a disproportionately high respiratory rate with less efficient ventilation throughout exercise and recovery, which will lead to higher-than-expected ventilatory equivalents (shown in Figure 9.3) with an RER >1.0.

VO_2 (and VCO_2) versus Work Rate versus Time Plot

All 9-panel plots contain a graph of VO_2 versus work rate (some also include a VCO_2 plot on the same graph for a better overall appreciation of exercise capacity).

Graph Notations

- A diagonal line may be included to show the predicted rate of increase in VO_2 for the work rate increase.

The increase in VO_2 relative to work rate ($\Delta VO_2/\Delta WR$) is dependent on the following:

- The ability of the cardiovascular system to deliver oxygenated arterial blood
- The ability of the musculature to extract oxygen from arterial blood.

$\Delta VO_2/\Delta WR$

- Sometimes referred to as work efficiency or response gain.
- It is a marker of O_2 transport and utilisation, and can give a global assessment of exercise capacity/tolerance and the presence of exercise limitation.
- The normal range is approximately 9–12 ml/min/watt.
- Is independent of sex, age, and height.
- Can also be assessed during submaximal exercise.

Normal Responses

- VO_2 should increase linearly during exercise with a similar gradient to work rate (i.e. in parallel) as shown in Figure 10.1.
- Beyond the AT, VO_2 becomes cardiac output dependent.

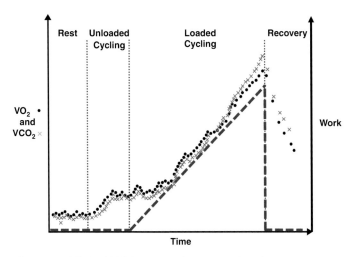

Figure 10.1 VO$_2$ (and VCO$_2$) versus work rate versus time plot

Variations or Abnormal Responses

- Shallow gradient $\Delta VO_2/\Delta WR$ slope
  - Implies that VO$_2$ is unable to match increasing work rate and usually represents reduced O$_2$ transport due to a cardiovascular limitation or peripheral vascular disease (reduced O$_2$ delivery to legs).
- Other less common causes include the following:
  - Reduced or abnormal O$_2$ utilisation, for example mitochondrial myopathy
  - Abnormal muscle oxygen metabolism, for example cystic fibrosis.

VCO₂ versus VO₂ Plot

- The anaerobic threshold (AT) is the point beyond which work is done by *both* a combination of aerobic *and* anaerobic metabolism.
- It is the point at which aerobic metabolism is supplemented by anaerobic metabolism.
- The first plot to examine is VCO_2 versus VO_2. The AT is the point at which the gradient of the curve changes and becomes steeper, as VCO_2 increases to a greater degree than VO_2 (shown in Figure 11.1).

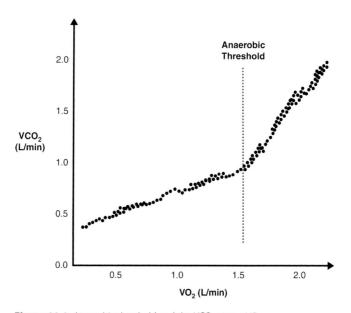

Figure 11.1 Anaerobic threshold and the VCO_2 versus VO_2

- Remember at this point that lactic acid production has increased, and the increase in H$^+$ ions is being buffered by HCO$^-_3$, resulting in more CO$_2$ being produced/exhaled.
- The AT can be derived by one of the following two methods:
- The V-slope method –
  - in this method the AT is taken as the inflection point where VCO$_2$ increases more than VO$_2$ (this increase in CO$_2$ production is eliminated by an increase in ventilation), shown in Figure 11.2.
- 'Line of One' or 'Line of Unity' method –
  - in this method, the breakpoint is determined by visual inspection using a line with a gradient of 1. This line is 'brought in' along the x-axis from right to left. The AT in this method is the tangential breakpoint in the VCO$_2$ versus VO$_2$ relationship – that is the first point that excess VCO$_2$ is evident, and the first point on the curve that touches the 'line of one', as shown in Figure 11.3.

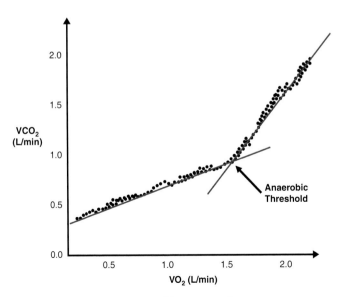

Figure 11.2 The V-slope method of determining AT

Interpreting a Cardiopulmonary Exercise Test

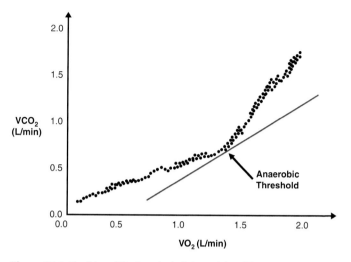

Figure 11.3 The 'Line of One' method of determining AT

Normal Responses

- It is generally accepted that an AT of >40% predicted max VO_2 is considered normal. If patients do not reach their max VO_2, figures may seem abnormally elevated (e.g. if AT is closer to VO_2 peak). Hence the importance of interpreting AT in terms of its absolute number as well as its percentage of max and peak VO_2. There is a wide range for normality (40–80%).
  - Trained athlete 61–80%
  - Normal 51–60%
  - Deconditioned/mild disease 41–50%
  - Abnormal <40%.

Variations or Abnormal Responses

The three main scenarios in which anaerobic metabolism supplements aerobic metabolism when supply fails to meet demands are as follows:

- Low cardiac output
- Obstructed leg blood vessels
- Low peripheral oxygen saturations.

VEVO$_2$ and VEVCO$_2$ versus Time (or Work or VO$_2$) Plot

- Ventilatory equivalents are unitless values that describe the ventilation (ml/min) required to either take up 1 ml of oxygen (ml/min) or eliminate 1 ml of carbon dioxide (ml/min).
- They act as an index of lung function, for example, inefficiency can be shown when there is high ventilation with poor O$_2$ uptake or CO$_2$ elimination.

Normal Responses

- At rest perfusion is markedly better at lung bases than at the apices. The anatomical dead space to resting tidal volume ratio is also greater.
- During exercise cardiac output increases, leading to increased apical perfusion recruiting previously under-perfused alveoli, resulting in better V/Q matching and a gradual fall in VEVO$_2$ and VEVCO$_2$ (shown in Figure 12.1).
- The nadir of VEVO$_2$ and VEVCO$_2$ shows the point of optimal lung function in terms of oxygenation and eliminating CO$_2$, respectively.
- If the lowest value for VEVCO$_2$ is >32, it implies a high physiological dead space fraction (a high VD/Vt ratio) – that there is inefficient ventilation/poor gas exchange, for example pulmonary vascular disease.
- A value of >34 has been associated with increased risk in the literature.

The Anaerobic Threshold

- As the test continues, VEVO$_2$ begins to suddenly increase at the AT (i.e. the nadir just *before* rise represents the AT) when ventilation must increase to remove CO$_2$ and buffer the lactic acidaemia.

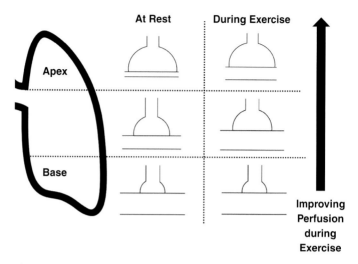

Figure 12.1 Ventilation/perfusion variations within the lungs at rest and during exercise

- However, VO_2 can't increase further, hence the sudden increase in ventilation per millilitre of O_2 – it doesn't represent a reduction in lung efficiency.

The Respiratory Compensation Point

- Like $VEVO_2$, $VEVCO_2$ starts to increase towards the end of exercise at the respiratory compensation point (RCP), beyond the AT.
- The nadir of $VEVCO_2$ is not as distinct as that of $VEVO_2$ – tending to be more of a gradual curve (shown in Figure 12.2).
- The RCP is not always seen during CPET. The presence of the RCP indicates that the patient has developed a sufficient lactate to become acidaemic and that ventilation is *not* limited by exercise (i.e. good effort).
- In patients with lung disease, ventilation is limited by exercise capacity, so there is no ability to increase ventilation to compensate for acidaemia and there is no RCP.

VEVO$_2$ and VEVCO$_2$ versus Time (or Work or VO$_2$) Plot

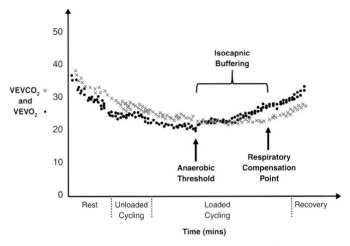

Figure 12.2 AT, RCP, and Isocapnic buffering on the VEVO$_2$ and VEVCO$_2$ versus time curve

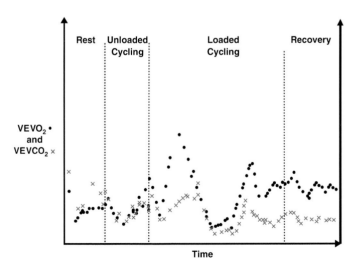

Figure 12.3 Dysfunctional breathing on the VEVO$_2$ versus VEVCO$_2$ versus time plot

Isocapnic Buffering

- The time period between the AT and the RCP represents the period that lactic acid is buffered by HCO_3^- (shown in Figure 12.2).

Variations or Abnormal Responses

- High $VEVCO_2$ (at AT or slope) implies the following:
  - ○ An increase in physiological dead space fraction (indicating reduced gas exchange efficiency)
  - ○ Reduced $PaCO_2$ (e.g. as a result of hyperventilation).
- $VEVCO_2$ is elevated in heart failure, pulmonary disease, and pulmonary hypertension, and can be used as a predictive marker of disease progression, morbidity, and mortality.
- Dysfunctional/Oscillatory breathing and hyperventilation can be seen by highly variable and irregular $VEVCO_2$, as shown in Figure 12.3.

PETO$_2$ and PETCO$_2$ versus Time (or Work or VO$_2$) Plot

This plot examines the end-tidal partial pressures of O$_2$ and CO$_2$ (the plot may also include arterial partial pressures if invasive monitoring is also used).

- Normally they will look like mirror images of each other (with O$_2$ plotted above CO$_2$), shown in Figure 13.1.
- The magnitude of changes depends on the RER.

Normal ResponsesEnd-Tidal O$_2$

- At the start of exercise end-tidal O$_2$ levels will gradually fall as a greater amount of O$_2$ is extracted from inspired air, leaving less in expired air.

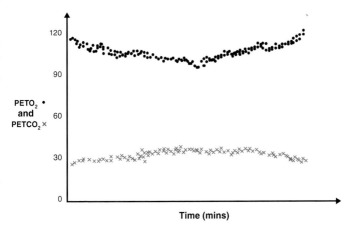

Figure 13.1 PETO$_2$ and PETCO$_2$ versus time (or work) plot

- Beyond the AT, ventilation increases without an increase in VO_2, hence the end-tidal O_2 increases to resemble inspired air again.

End-Tidal CO_2

- At the start of exercise, end-tidal CO_2 levels will gradually rise due to increased production.
- At the RCP, ventilation increases due to acidaemia and end-tidal CO_2 begins to fall.

Anaerobic Threshold

- The AT is seen at the nadir of $PETO_2$ (plateau or falling), that is $PETO_2$ must *not* be rising.
- For $PETCO_2$, the AT is seen when $P_{ET}CO_2$ plateaus and is not falling, whereas the respiratory compensation point is the point at which $PETCO_2$ begins to fall (see Figure 13.2). The section of the curve between these two points represents isocapnic buffering.

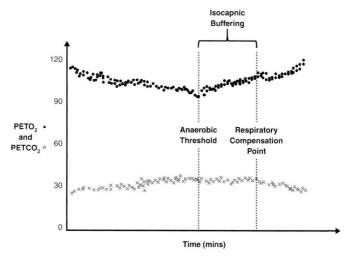

Figure 13.2 AT and RCP on the $PETO_2$ and $PETCO_2$ versus time (or work) plot

Variations or Abnormal Responses

- Low PETCO$_2$ implies either hyperventilation or high V/Q ratio (i.e. high dead space).
- Checking against RER can help determine whether hyperventilation is acute or chronic (this can be corroborated by arterial blood gas analysis or knowledge of plasma HCO$_3^-$).

Heart Rate and O_2 Pulse (VO_2/HR) versus Time Plot

Heart rate should steadily increase with exercise and is normally the factor that limits exercise capacity.

- Maximum HR (bpm) = 220 − age
  - Therefore, maximum HR decreases with advancing age.
  - Normal = >85% predicted.
- Heart rate reserve (HRR) – the ability to increase HR further at peak exercise (shown in Figure 14.1).
  - HRR = predicted HR_{max} − observed HR_{max}.

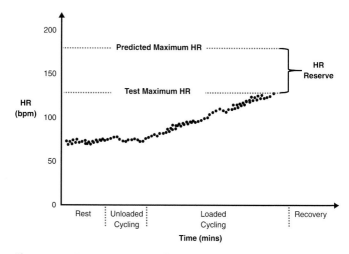

Figure 14.1 Heart rate reserve on the HR versus time plot

○ %HRR used $= [(\mathrm{HR_{peak}} - \mathrm{HR_{rest}})/(220 - \mathrm{age} - \mathrm{HR_{rest}})] \times 100$.
○ Used to estimate the 'stress' on the cardiovascular system during exercise.
○ Normal = zero or <15–20%.

Potential reasons for not reaching predicted max HR (and therefore having a higher heart rate reserve) can include the following:
- Normal interpatient variability
- Poor effort
- Use of negative chronotropic drugs (e.g. beta-blockers)
- Disease processes (e.g. heart, lung, peripheral vascular, musculoskeletal, etc.).

Normal Responses

- Heart rate will steadily (and linearly) increase with exercise to >85% predicted HRmax.
  ○ That is, a low HRR is normal.

Variations or Abnormal Responses

- Failure of HR to rise (chronotropic insufficiency) is seen in patients using negatively chronotropic drugs (e.g. beta-blockers), SA node dysfunction and autonomic dysfunction (e.g. in diabetes).
- A non-linear increase in HR can be seen when there is an increased rate of HR response. This usually occurs when either stroke volume is reduced or the maximal stroke volume is reached early (due to pathology).

Low Heart Rate Reserve

- This is usually normal; however, it may be abnormal in certain scenarios.
- For example, it can be seen in unfit patients or those with impaired ventricular function (with or without pulmonary vascular resistance), where increasing cardiac output relies on increasing heart rate (rather than stroke volume). This often results in a rapid rise in HR coupled with a low VO_2 max. Often these patients will have a high resting HR as part of physiological compensation (possibly with high sympathetic tone, in the absence of beta-blockade).

High Heart Rate Reserve

- This is seen when HRmax is less than 85% predicted.
- There are several potential causes, including the following:
  - Poor effort
  - Chronotropic insufficiency, for example sick sinus syndrome or beta-blockade
  - Angina that limits exercise
  - Lung disease resulting in a prematurely ending test
  - Peripheral vascular disease with claudication resulting in a prematurely ending test.

Oxygen Pulse

- Oxygen pulse (ml/beat) is oxygen uptake (VO_2) in ml/min divided by heart rate (in bpm).
  - O_2 pulse $= VO_2/HR$.
- Reflects the volume of oxygen taken into blood (VO_2) up by lungs per heartbeat.
- We know that cardiac output is the product of HR and stroke volume (SV).
  - $CO = SV \times HR$.

- By using this, together with the Fick principle, we can rearrange and use O_2 pulse as an indirect/non-invasive surrogate indicator of stroke volume.
  - $CO = VO_2/[CaO_2 - CvO_2]$.
  - Rearrange to
    - $VO_2 = CO \times [CaO_2 - CvO_2]$.
  - Hence
    - $VO_2 = [SV \times HR] \times [CaO_2 - CvO_2]$,
  where
    - $CaO_2 = 1.34 \times Hb \times SaO_2 + (0.0031 \times PaO_2)$,
    - $CvO_2 = 1.34 \times Hb \times SvO_2 + (0.0031 \times PvO_2)$.
- If we assume the arteriovenous difference ($CaO_2 - CvO_2$) to remain relatively constant, we can rearrange to
    - O_2 pulse $= VO_2/HR \approx SV$.
    - However, it is important to consider potential causes of reduced arterial oxygen content and altered oxygen extraction when interpreting O_2 pulse.

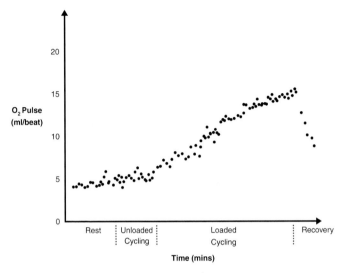

Heart Rate and O_2 Pulse (VO_2/HR) versus Time Plot

O₂ Pulse (ml/beat) axis: 0, 5, 10, 15, 20

Time axis labels: Rest | Unloaded Cycling | Loaded Cycling | Recovery

Time (mins)

Figure 14.2 O_2 pulse (VO_2/HR) versus time plot

Normal Responses

- O_2 pulse will increase in linear fashion with increasing VO_2 and increasing heart rate (reflecting increasing stroke volume).
- As exercise continues, the rate of increase in O_2 pulse slows.
- This is because the continued increase in VO_2 (and cardiac output) is more due to increasing HR than increasing SV, as shown in Figure 14.2.
- Hence, in most cases, plateauing or falling O_2 pulse is abnormal and indicates maximal SV.
- However, it is possible that a high O_2 pulse plateau may be normal in trained athletes who are performing near maximal exercise capacity.
- Predicted O_2 pulse = predicted VO_2 max/predicted HR max
  - Normal = 80% predicted or >10 ml/beat.
- Trained athletes are able to achieve a very high O_2 pulse due to the ability to increase stroke volume whilst maintaining a relatively lower heart rate, and that increased oxygen extraction is due to increased mitochondrial density and myoglobin levels.

Variations or Abnormal Responses

- It is important to check whether a patient has any reason for rate limitation (e.g. beta-blockade).
- Low O_2 pulse is usually a marker of cardiac disease.
- Causes of low O_2 pulse include the following:
  ○ Low level of cardiorespiratory fitness
  ○ Prematurely ending test not due to cardiovascular disease, for example knee pain
  ○ Reduced haemoglobin (and therefore, oxygen content), for example anaemia or carboxyhaemoglobinaemia
  ○ Reduced blood oxygenation in the lungs
  ○ Right-to-left shunt
  ○ Reduced peripheral oxygen extraction and mitochondrial dysfunction (as seen in jaundice, post-chemotherapy, and metabolic disorders).
- Causes of high O_2 pulse include the following:
  ○ High level of cardiorespiratory fitness
  ○ Use of negatively chronotropic drugs (e.g. beta-blockade).
- In heart disease, stroke volume changes may be limited (it may not change at all), and cardiac output increases can only be achieved by increasing heart rate.
- A sudden drop or early plateau in O_2 pulse may indicate the development of cardiac ischaemia or a fixed SV (as seen in aortic stenosis or left-ventricular outflow tract obstruction). There is often a corresponding increase in the rate of HR increase, with a break point in HR response indicating the compensation for reduced SV.

Heart Rate Recovery

- Heart rate recovery is the rate of decline in heart rate after the cessation of exercise.
- Normally measured after the first minute of recovery.
- Heart rate recovery (usually expressed as a percentage) is derived as

$$(\text{Max observed HR} - \text{HR at 1 minute during recovery})/100.$$

- Heart rate recovery is considered normal if HR falls by >10% within 1 minute during recovery.
- Reflects the state of the autonomic nervous systems and its effect on the cardiovascular system.

- Delayed or prolonged heart rate recovery implies abnormal autonomic regulation and increased cardiac risk. Causes can include the following:
  - Decreased vagal or parasympathetic tone
  - Increased sympathetic activation
  - Abnormal cardiopulmonary baroreflexes.

VE versus Time Plot

Minute ventilation (VE) is the sum of the volumes of each breath over the course of a minute.

- Depends on respiratory rate and tidal volume.
- VE_{max} is measured during CPET; however, it can also be predicted.
- Predicted maximum minute ventilation (VE_{max}) can theoretically be estimated using FEV_1 (measured in litres).
  - Predicted $VE_{max}(L/min) = (FEV_1 \times 20) + 20$.

Maximum Voluntary Ventilation

- A measure of maximal breathing capacity.
- Assessed by measuring the maximum airflow, at rest, over a 12–15-second period.
  - This involves a form of hyperventilation, which is not recommended before cardiopulmonary exercise testing.
- Approximated by $MVV = FEV_1 \times 40$.
  - This is calculated by software. It is important to measure the actual FEV_1, otherwise the software will use predicted FEV_1 and may lead to error.
- May be included as either a horizontal or a vertical annotation of ventilatory curves.

Breathing Reserve

- Also called 'ventilatory reserve'.
- This describes the relationship between the minute ventilation seen during exercise and the predicted maximal breathing capacity (as estimated by the maximum voluntary ventilation (MVV)) – usually expressed as a percentage or in absolute terms.

- $BR = 100(MVV - VE_{max})/MVV$.
- Alternatively, $BR = [1 - (VE_{max}/MVV)] \times 100$.
- That is, breathing reserve is the % of MVV not used at peak exercise.
- Normal, healthy, non-athlete subjects will have breathing reserve (BR) $\geq 30\%$ or 15 L/min (i.e. they use $<70\%$ of their MVV at maximal exertion (shown in Figure 15.1).
- Cardiac patients may have a normal BR.
- Lung disease patients will likely have little to no BR at peak exercise.
  - That is, VE_{max} is $>70\%$ predicted with low BR $<30\%$, meaning that there is little possibility of increasing ventilation any further.

Normal Responses

- Minute ventilation (VE) increases with exercise and workload (shown in Figure 15.1).
- VE does not normally limit exercise.
- Exercise tends to be limited by cardiac output (in healthy subjects and those with cardiac disease).

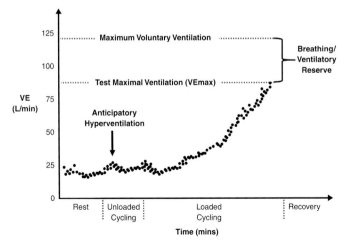

Figure 15.1 Normal VE versus time plot and breathing/ventilatory reserve

- Hence, VE_{max} does not reach 70% predicted and there is a high ventilatory reserve.

Variations/Abnormal Responses

- Exercise is not normally limited by ventilation.
- Patients with lung disease may have a low breathing reserve (<30%, meaning that VE_{max} is >70% predicted).
- If peak VO_2 is low and the subject stops due to ventilatory limitation (VE_{max} >70%), it is likely that their HR will be <85% predicted maximum.
- That is, it may appear as if the test has ended prematurely, before maximum capacity has been reached.

Dysfunctional (Oscillatory) Breathing

- Erratic ventilation (not necessarily due to lung disease) can be implied by an erratic VE throughout CPET (shown in Figure 15.2).

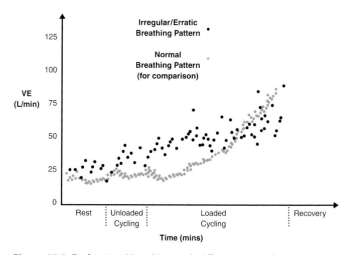

Figure 15.2 Dysfunctional breathing on the VE versus time plot

VE versus VCO_2 Plot

This plot examines the link between alveolar minute ventilation and VCO_2, which is usually tightly matched, and is an alternative means of viewing the relationship previously shown on the VEVCO$_2$ versus time plot.

- The linear portion of the curve before the respiratory compensation point is used to assess lung efficiency.
- A gradient of >32 implies inefficient ventilation (i.e. an inability to clear CO_2, which may be cardiac or respiratory in origin; this should be checked against the Vt versus VE curve).
- High VE with low VCO_2 implies poor lung function.
- Ventilatory equivalents are another way of assessing lung efficiency.

Normal Responses

- Minute ventilation (VE) increases with exercise along with carbon dioxide production (VCO_2).
- Hence the plot should be linear.
- Beyond the AT, lactate accumulation results in an acidaemia.
- This is initially compensated for by HCO_3^- (isocapnic buffering).
- However, at the respiratory compensation point (RCP), this buffering capacity is exceeded and acidaemia is then buffered by increasing ventilation to clear CO_2, as shown in Figure 16.1.
- By driving down $PaCO_2$, the diffusion gradient across alveoli is reduced; hence less CO_2 is exhaled, resulting in a steepening of the gradient of the slope. A phenomenon that is mirrored in the $PETO_2$ and $PETCO_2$ versus time plot as a fall in $PETCO_2$ after the respiratory compensation point, also shown in Figure 16.1.

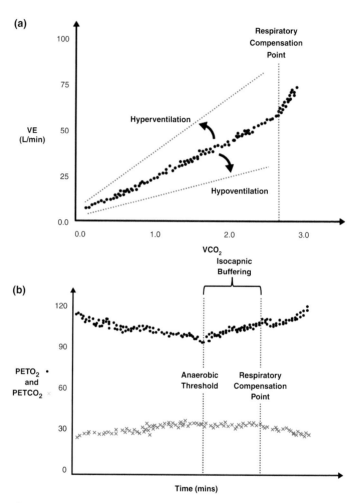

Figure 16.1 VE versus VCO_2 plot (a) and $PETO_2$ and $PETCO_2$ versus time plot (b)

Variations or Abnormal Responses

- Shallow VE versus VCO_2 slope gradient is seen in health, but may be seen in CO_2 retention or hypoventilation.
- Steep VE versus VCO_2 slope gradient implies:

- ○ V/Q mismatch with increased dead space/tidal volume ratio (VD/Vt)
- ○ Hyperventilation/low PaCO$_2$ (e.g. low driving pressure to remove CO$_2$ into alveolar gas, as seen in heart failure).
- This has been shown to be an independent risk factor for morbidity and mortality in perioperative, cardiac, and respiratory literature.

Vt versus VE Plot

This plot examines the relationship between tidal volume (Vt) and minute ventilation (VE).

- The curves may include dashed lines that intersect axes to represent additional parameters.
  - Y-axis – vital (VC) and inspiratory capacities (IC)
  - X-axis – maximum voluntary ventilation (MVV).

- Breathing or ventilatory reserve (BR) can be illustrated as shown in Figure 17.1.

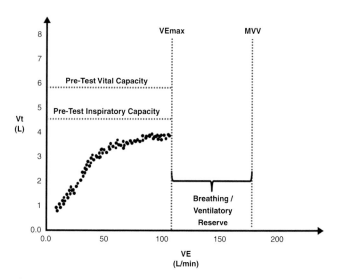

Figure 17.1 BR and MVV on the Vt versus VE plot

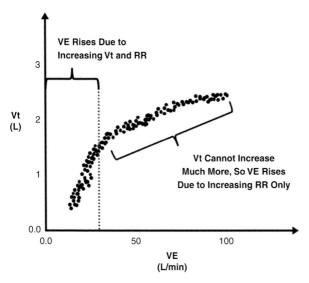

Figure 17.2 Normal Vt versus VE plot

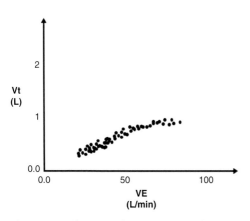

Figure 17.3 Obstructive disease pattern on the Vt versus VE plot

Normal Responses

- The normal shape of the curve is a 'dogleg' or building up to a plateau.
- At low-intensity exercise, VE increases mainly due to increasing tidal volume.
- As intensity increases, further increases in VE are achieved by increasing respiratory rate, whilst Vt tends to plateau as shown in Figure 17.2.

Variations or Abnormal Responses

- Patients with lung disease rely on increasing respiratory rate (as they are unable to increase their tidal volume to a great degree) and have flatter curves, reaching a plateau earlier, as shown in Figure 17.3.
- A shallow, flatter curve implies obstructive disease.
- A steep curve approaching inspiratory capacity implies restrictive disease.

Chapter 18

Additional Parameters of Interest and Presentation of Results

There are several other parameters that can influence our interpretation of a CPET. These include the following:

- Oxygen saturation (SpO_2)
- Oxygen uptake efficiency slope (OUES)
- Alveolar-arterial PO_2 pressure difference and PaO_2
- Physiologic dead space-to-tidal volume ratio (VD/Vt).

We have opted not to include the latter two parameters as they require peri-procedural blood sampling to provide accurate results and are beyond the scope of this text. It is worth noting that several manufacturers of CPET software may include VD/Vt as part of their calculations from gas analysis, and to be aware that this measurement is not accurate and therefore cannot be relied upon.

Oxygen Saturation (SpO_2)

- Pulse oximeters form part of the standard monitoring equipment used during CPET.
- They operate by detecting the differences in the absorption of two different wavelengths of light passing between a light-emitting diode and a photodetector on a probe (usually placed on a finger or ear) as blood flows through pulsating vessels.
- Oxygenated and deoxygenated blood absorb light at different wavelengths and the amount absorbed varies as vessels expand and contract with the pulse (according to Beer–Lambert law). The ratio of these absorption amplitudes is then used to estimate arterial O_2 saturation.

  ○ However, pulse oximeters do not measure or estimate the arterial partial pressure of oxygen (PaO_2), which can decrease to a large degree whilst SpO_2 remains relatively unchanged, due to the shape of the oxy-haemoglobin dissociation curve (shown in Figure 18.1).

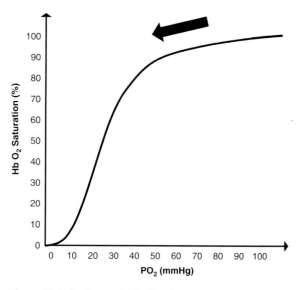

Figure 18.1 Oxy-haemoglobin dissociation curve

- When compared to directly measured arterial O_2 saturation, pulse oximeters with a good signal are reasonably accurate with 95% confidence intervals of ±4–5%.
- However, there are several factors than can affect accuracy, including the following:
  ○ SpO_2 <88%
  ○ Dark skin pigmentation
  ○ Poor peripheral perfusion
  ○ The presence of carboxyhaemoglobin or methaemoglobin
  ○ Movement artefact.

Normal Responses
- SpO_2 should remain relatively constant throughout exercise.

Variations or Abnormal Responses
- In the absence of known lung disease, a fall in SpO_2 of greater than 4–5% from the resting value is unusual and may imply significant pathology. Causes include the following:
- Artefact

- Poor signal, for example movement, gripping handlebars too tightly, and so on.
- Impaired diffusion
  - At rest red blood cells (RBCs) spend approximately 0.75 seconds within pulmonary capillaries. Within 0.25 seconds Hb is fully saturated with oxygen (as shown in Figure 18.2).
  - Thickening of the alveolar membrane (e.g. pulmonary fibrosis) slows O_2 diffusion and prevents PaO_2 equilibrating with PAO_2.
  - Exercise increases pulmonary blood flow, and RBCs can spend as little as 0.25 seconds in pulmonary capillaries. When combined with diffusion limitation, hypoxaemia can result.
- V/Q mismatch
  - In patients with pulmonary vascular disease, there may not be the capacity to accommodate increased blood volume during exercise. This results in blood being diverted to other areas of the lungs, resulting in congestion or over-perfusion and hypoxaemia.
- Right-to-left cardiac shunt
  - During exercise, right heart pressure increases and any previously undiagnosed atrial septal defect (e.g. patent foramen ovale) may open, resulting in a right-to-left shunt in which

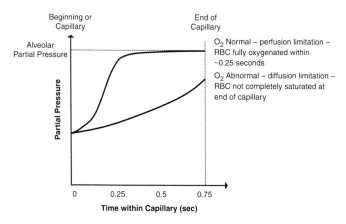

Figure 18.2 Variation of the partial pressure of oxygen during red blood cell (RBC) transit within pulmonary capillaries

deoxygenated blood bypasses the lungs, crossing from the right to the left side of the heart, mixing with oxygenated blood that is pumped into the systemic circulation. This reduces the overall oxygen content of blood leaving the left heart, resulting in hypoxaemia.

Oxygen Uptake Efficiency Slope

- The OUES aims to demonstrate the relationship between oxygen uptake and total ventilation and has been shown to strongly correlate with VO_2.
- It is an independent and objective measure of cardiopulmonary reserve requiring only submaximal exercise; thus it can be useful in patients unable to complete a maximal test.
- This is achieved by the use of a slope of the regression line on semi-logarithmic plot of VO_2 versus logVE (shown in Figure 18.3).
- This is not usually part of the standard 9-panel plot.
- Oxygen uptake efficiency slope is influenced by the following:
  - VCO_2, which is determined by aerobic metabolism in muscle and bicarbonate buffering
  - Arterial pCO_2
  - Physiological dead space ventilation.

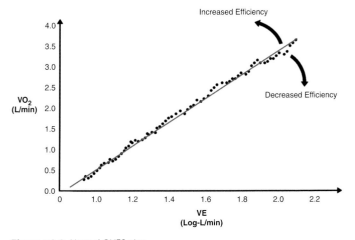

Figure 18.3 Normal OUES plot

- A steeper slope (higher OUES) represents increased efficiency in oxygen delivery (i.e. ventilation easily matches oxygen uptake).
- A shallower slope (lower OUES) represents decreased efficiency in oxygen delivery (i.e. higher ventilation is needed for a given oxygen uptake), which can be seen in the following:
  - Advancing age is associated with a gradual decline in OUES
  - Increased physiological dead space ventilation, for example smokers, lung disease, and pulmonary vascular disease
  - Cardiac limitation
  - Deconditioning.
- Predicted values can be calculated by using reference equations from Hollenburg and Tager (2000), measured in ml/min/log (L/min).
  - For males
    - $\text{OUES} = [1320 - (26.7 \times \text{age}) + (1394 \times \text{BSA})]$
      - BSA is the body surface area.
  - For females
    - $\text{OUES} = [1175 - (15.8 \times \text{age}) + (841 \times \text{BSA})]$.

  Alternatively, equations from Sun ct al. (2012) can be used to provide OUES in L/min/log(L/min):
  - For males
    - $-1.178 - (\text{age} \times 0.032) + (0.023 \times \text{height(cm)}) + (0.008 \times \text{weight(kg)})$.
  - For females
    - $-0.61 - (\text{age} \times 0.032) + (0.023 \times \text{height(cm)}) + (0.008 \times \text{weight(kg)})$.

Chronotropic Index

- Chronotropic index (CI) is sometimes used to describe two different phenomena:
  - The % of heart rate reserve (HRR) used, as defined by the following formula:
    - $\text{CI} = [(\text{HR}_{peak} - \text{HR}_{rest})/(220 - \text{age} - \text{HR}_{rest})] \times 100$.

- - This is predominately used in cardiological stress tests.
  - Chronotropic index <80% usually suggests either chronotropic insufficiency/incompetence (which may be due to heart failure, arrhythmia, or drug related, e.g. beta-blockers) or a submaximal test (e.g. respiratory limitation or joint pain terminating test).
  - ○ The relationship between HR and VO_2, which we will discuss further.
- From the Fick equation we know that VO_2 depends on cardiac output, and that cardiac output is the product of heart rate and stroke volume.
- Normally, this results in a linear relationship, the slope of which is the CI (as shown in Figure 18.4). Chronotropic index is calculated using the following formula:

$$CI = \left[\frac{PeakHR - RestingHR}{PredictedHR - RestingHR} \right] \Big/ \left[\frac{(PeakVO_2 - RestingVO_2)}{PredictedVO_2 - RestingVO_2} \right]$$

- This is distinct from the oxygen pulse, which is the relationship between HR and VO_2 at a moment in time.
- The normal range is 0.8–1.3.
- A CI of 1.0 indicates that HR increases in-line with VO_2.
- Chronotropic index >1.0 indicates that the HR is increasing more rapidly than VO_2.
  - ○ Can be seen with deconditioning or cardiac limitation.

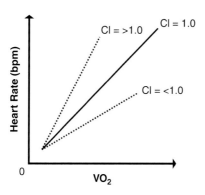

Figure 18.4 Chronotropic index

- Chronotropic index <1.0 indicates that HR is increasing more slowly than VO_2.
  - Can be seen in chronotropic insufficiency.
  - Can also be seen in trained athletes (although these individuals usually have a supra-normal peak VO_2).

Presentation of Results

A cardiopulmonary exercise test report should include the following:
- The reason for the referral
- Patient background information (including history of the presenting complaint, past medical history, drug history, and exercise history for example normal activity, any limitations, any changes in the recent past)
- The data from the cardiopulmonary exercise test (at minimum this should include the raw data set, and ideally should also include a copy of the 9-panel plot)
- A summary of the test highlighting:
  - Overall exercise capacity/cardiopulmonary fitness
  - The presence and likely cause of any exercise limitation or abnormal responses
  - If being used in the peri-operative setting – an estimation of peri-operative risk (morbidity and mortality) – suggestions for optimisation or further investigation and potential level of post-operative care (e.g. ward-level care or enhanced care on a high-dependency or intensive care unit) should be included.

In terms of CPET raw data, we would suggest including the following as a minimum:
- Baseline observations and relevant investigations or results (e.g. HR, Resting ECG, BP, SpO_2, Height, Weight, BMI, and Hb level)
- Incremental test gradient (in watts/min)
- Phase durations: rest, unloaded, loaded, and recovery
- Patient effort/test quality (maximal, submaximal, or poor effort)
- Reason for stopping (e.g. leg fatigue, shortness of breath, or knee pain)
- Any issues during the test or recovery phases (e.g. issues with pedal cadence or other compliance issues and ECG/BP/SpO_2 changes)
- Spirometry (FEV1, FVC, and FEV1/FVC)
- CPET parameters – (measured, predicted, and % predicted values, and an indication of whether low/normal/high)

- Maximum work
- METS
- RER at peak exercise
- Peak VO_2 (+/– comparison with OUES if test was submaximal)
- AT
- VO_2/WR slope
- O_2 pulse
- Peak HR
- Heart rate reserve
- Heart rate recovery
- $VEVCO_2$ (at AT and slope)
- Breathing reserve.

Chapter

General Interpretation and a Normal Test

19

There are many different potential causes of exercise limitation and there can be overlap between disease processes. We suggest applying the approach to interpretation outlined in Table 8.1 and Figure 8.7, explore what constitutes a 'normal' test, and how parameters may vary in different clinical scenarios.

- We need to understand what a normal test looks like in order to identify potential abnormal physiology or disease. See Figure 19.1, Table 19.1, and Figure 19.2.

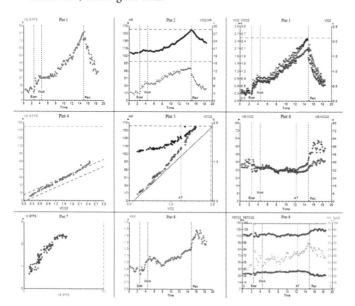

Figure 19.1 Normal CPET: Wasserman plot

Table 19.1 Normal CPET parameters

Exercise parameters	Test result	Normal range
Maximum work	156 watts (90%)	>80% predicted
METS	5.4 (82%)	>80% predicted
RER at peak exercise	1.19	>1.15
Cardiopulmonary parameters		
Peak VO_2	18.9 ml/min/kg (82%)	>80% predicted
VO_2 at AT	14.7 ml/min/kg (78%)	>40% predicted VO_2 peak
VO_2/WR slope	9.8	9–12 and linear
VO_2/HR – oxygen pulse	13 ml/beat (83%)	>80% predicted
Peak HR	159 bpm (98%)	>85% predicted
Heart rate reserve	<20%	<20%
Heart rate recovery	>10% peak HR at 1 minute	>10% peak HR at 1 minute
$VEVCO_2$ (at AT/ slope)	30	<32
Breathing reserve	58%	>30%
SpO_2	>95%	>95%

- It is tempting to simply call a test 'normal' if the patient's effort is maximal and the peak VO_2 is greater than 80% predicted. However, it is essential to review each parameter individually and to approach the test holistically to ensure that no subtle changes are missed and that graph patterns and values are within normal limits.

Test Review and Interpretation

- Was the patient's effort maximal?
  - Yes. The RER is >1.15, maximal work was >80% predicted, and maximum heart rate was >85% predicted.

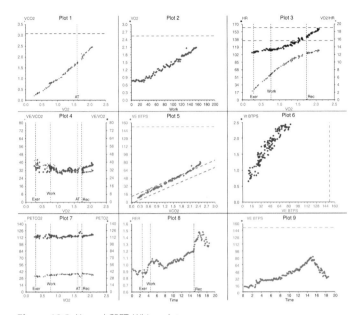

Figure 19.2 Normal CPET: Whipp plot

- Is the patient's exercise capacity normal?
  - Yes. Peak VO_2 is >80% predicted and the VO_2/WR slope is normal.
- When does anaerobic metabolism begin?
  - The AT is appropriate both in absolute terms and being >40% of the predicted VO_2.
- Is circulation or oxygen transport normal?
  - Yes. Oxygen pulse, peak HR, HR reserve, HR recovery, and $VEVCO_2$ are all within the normal range.
- Is ventilation or V/Q matching normal?
  - Yes. $VEVCO_2$, breathing reserve and SpO_2 are all within the normal range.
- Is the mechanism of exercise limitation visible and does it make sense with the clinical picture?
  - This is a normal test with good effort, no obvious exercise limitation, in a patient with normal cardiopulmonary fitness.

Chapter 20
Submaximal Test

- A submaximal test is a CPET in which the patient has been unable to achieve a peak exercise response, and is usually evidenced by failure to achieve the following:
  - RER <1.15
  - Maximal work <80% predicted
  - Maximal heart rate <85% predicted.

- As a consequence, the following can also be seen:
  - Peak VO_2 lower than predicted
  - Normal AT
  - No RCP
  - High heart rate reserve
  - High breathing reserve.

- The results of a submaximal test need to be interpreted with caution, taking into account the whole picture and trying to determine what limited exercise, for example pathology, pain, or enthusiasm.

  - This is because it is possible for a patient to perform 'maximally' without achieving an RER >1.15, with a lower work rate and reduced peak VO_2 due to pathological exercise limitation.
  - This is different to a patient who stops early without achieving an RER >1.15 due to knee pain. Hence the need for context.

- There are, however, certain parameters which are unaffected or can still be of use in submaximal situations, including the following:
  - OUES
  - $VEVCO_2$ slope.

- The reasons for a submaximal test need to be explored. We can broadly categorise them as follows:
  - Volitional, that is patient stops of their own volition, which may be due to anxiety, poor motivation, and so on
  - Non-volitional, for example pain preventing continuation or respiratory limitation and reduced breathing reserve.

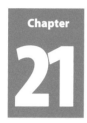

CPET in Trained Athletes, Deconditioning, and Obesity

Trained Athletes

- It is usually clear from the patient's exercise and past medical history if they possess a high level of cardiopulmonary fitness.
- In healthy, highly trained individuals, CPET parameters will often be supra-normal. Tests with 'just normal' results may indicate pathology in these patients.
- CPET in these healthy, fit patients usually shows:
  ○ Maximum work and METS >80% predicted
  ○ RER >1.15
  ○ Peak VO_2 greater than predicted
  ○ AT >60% predicted Peak VO_2
  ○ Peak VO_2/HR (oxygen pulse) greater than predicted (flattening is potentially normal at peak exercise)
  ○ Low resting heart rate
  ○ Low heart rate reserve
  ○ $VECO_2$ at AT (nadir) or slope <30
  ○ Clear respiratory compensation point
  ○ Breathing reserve can be <30% in the context of high Peak VO_2.

Obesity

- There is a spectrum of performance when it comes to testing patients living with obesity. Some are able to perform adequately and generate appropriate exercise responses, while others show evidence of deconditioning and potential signs of cardiorespiratory disease.
- This patient group can show different results depending on the type of ergometer used; additional patient effort is required when

using a treadmill when compared to a cycle ergometer, the latter only requiring leg rather than whole body movement.

- In the absence of cardiopulmonary disease, CPET in these patients usually shows the following:
  - Normal RER (>1.15) provided good motivation
  - Normal or slightly reduced peak VO_2 (may be lower when adjusted for body weight)
  - Normal or low/reduced AT (<40% predicted Peak VO_2)
  - Low heart rate reserve
  - Breathing reserve >30%
  - SpO_2 may be low at rest, improving during exercise.

Deconditioning

- This is a term used to describe inefficient delivery or use of oxygen at a tissue level.
- It is usually the result of a lack of regular exercise. However, patients with other pathology can also become concurrently deconditioned (e.g. peripheral vascular disease).
- The result profile in these patients is broadly similar to those patients with early cardiovascular disease or mild myopathies, as always evidence for corroborating signs, symptoms, and findings should be sought.
- CPET in these patients usually shows the following:

  - Reduced maximum workload with normal pattern on graphs
  - RER can be >1.15 or may be reduced when coupled with submaximal effort
  - Reduced peak VO_2
  - Normal or low/reduced AT (in absolute terms of <40% predicted Peak VO_2)
  - Oxygen pulse can be reduced
  - Low heart rate reserve
  - Breathing reserve >20%
  - Other cardiovascular, ventilatory, and gas exchange parameters tend to be normal. A typical CPET for a patient with deconditioning is shown in Figures 21.1 and 21.2 and Table 21.1 and described in 'Test review and interpretation'.

Table 21.1 Deconditioning CPET parameters

Exercise parameters	Test result	Normal range
Maximum work	82 watts (74%)	>80% predicted
METS	4.9 (70%)	>80% predicted
RER at peak exercise	1.33	>1.15
Cardiopulmonary parameters		
Peak VO_2	17.0 ml/min/kg (70%)	>80% predicted
VO_2 at AT	9.9 ml/min/kg (58%)	>40% predicted VO_2 peak
VO_2/WR slope	9.11	9–12 and linear
VO_2/HR – Oxygen pulse	8 ml/beat (71%)	>80% predicted
Peak HR	147 bpm (98%)	>85% predicted
Heart rate reserve	<20%	<20%
Heart rate recovery	>10% peak HR at 1 minute	>10% peak HR at 1 minute
$VEVCO_2$ (at AT/ slope)	34	<32
Breathing reserve	39%	>30%
SpO_2	>95%	>95%

Test Review and Interpretation

- Was the patient's effort maximal?
  - Potentially, but needs to be interpreted with caution.
  - The RER is >1.15 and maximal heart rate is >85% predicted; however, maximal work was <80% predicted.
- Is the patient's exercise capacity normal?
  - No, peak VO_2 is <80% predicted.
  - However, the VO_2/WR slope is normal, suggesting that exercise ability is potentially unaffected.

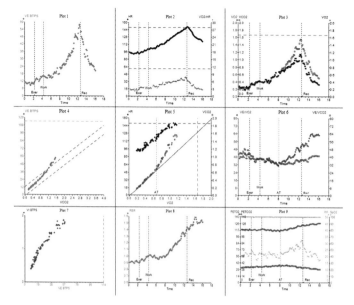

Figure 21.1 Deconditioning CPET: Wasserman plot

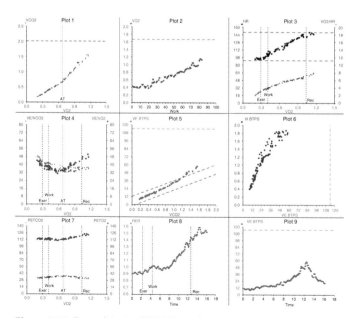

Figure 21.2 Deconditioning CPET: Whipp plot

- When does anaerobic metabolism begin?
  - The AT is low in absolute terms, despite being >40% of the predicted VO_2.
- Is circulation or oxygen transport normal?
  - Not entirely. Oxygen pulse is reduced (reflecting reduced peak VO_2).
  - However, peak HR, HR reserve, HR recovery, and $VEVCO_2$ are all within the normal range.
- Is ventilation or V/Q matching normal?
  - Not entirely. $VEVCO_2$ is marginally elevated at 34. However, breathing reserve and SpO_2 are all within the normal range.
- Is the mechanism of exercise limitation visible and does it make sense with the clinical picture?
  - This test shows reduced cardiopulmonary fitness, which is likely the result of deconditioning, as evidenced by low peak VO_2, low AT with reduced O_2 pulse, but otherwise normal or near-normal parameters.

Chapter 22

Cardiovascular Limitation

- In terms of cardiovascular limitation that can be elucidated by CPET, we can broadly categorise as follows:
  - Pump insufficiency
  - Ischaemic insufficiency
  - Chronotropic insufficiency
    - Here, there is a failure of heart rate to rise as expected.
  - Oxygen carriage insufficiency
    - For example, anaemia.
  - Right-to-left intracardiac shunt
    - For example, patent foramen ovale (in which SpO_2 falls with exercise and oxygen pulse is lower than predicted).
- There are general parameters that suggest cardiovascular limitation, including the following:
  - Reduced maximum workload
  - Reduced peak VO_2
  - Low or reduced AT (in absolute terms or <40% predicted peak VO_2)
  - Reduced oxygen pulse, which may plateau
  - A rapid, early rise in heart rate
  - Low heart rate reserve
  - Elevated $VEVCO_2$.
- We'll explore this in more detail in the following two examples.

Example 1

A typical CPET for a patient with cardiovascular disease is shown in Figures 22.1 and 22.2 and Table 22.1 and described in 'Test Review and Interpretation'.

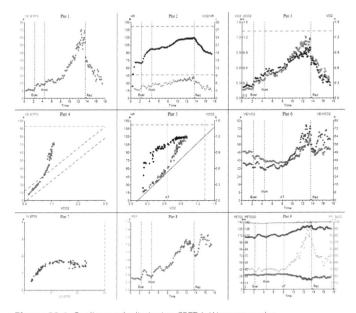

Figure 22.1 Cardiovascular limitation CPET 1: Wasserman plot

Test Review and Interpretation

- Was the patient's effort maximal?
  - Needs to be interpreted with caution.
  - The RER is >1.15.
  - However, maximal work was <80% predicted and maximum heart rate was <85% predicted.
- Is the patient's exercise capacity normal?
  - No. Peak VO_2 and maximum work are both reduced, indicating reduced exercise capacity.
  - However, the VO_2/WR slope is normal, suggesting that exercise ability is potentially unaffected.
- When does anaerobic metabolism begin?
  - The AT is low (in absolute terms) despite being >40% of the predicted VO_2.

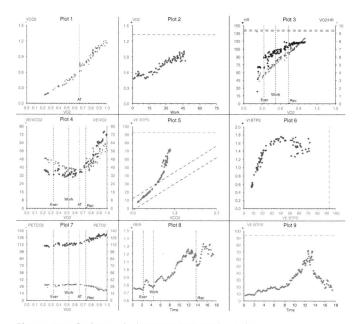

Figure 22.2 Cardiovascular limitation CPET 1: Whipp plot

- Is circulation or oxygen transport normal?
  - ○ Not entirely. The oxygen pulse has a consistently shallow gradient (Wasserman plot).
  - ○ Peak HR is <85% predicted and HR appears to plateau during exercise. HR recovery appears to be acceptable, whilst VEVCO$_2$ is elevated.

- Is ventilation or V/Q matching normal?
  - ○ Not entirely. SpO$_2$ remains normal throughout exercise and breathing reserve is just within the normal range.
  - ○ However, VEVCO2 slope and VEVCO2 at AT are both elevated. This could be cardiac in origin (due to increased dead space fraction), but ventilatory or pulmonary vascular limitation are also possible, which needs further investigation.

Table 22.1 Cardiovascular limitation CPET 1 parameters

Exercise parameters	Test result	Normal range
Maximum work	46 watts (57%)	>80% predicted
METS	4.7 (76%)	>80% predicted
RER at peak exercise	1.16	>1.15
Cardiopulmonary parameters		
Peak VO_2	16.4 ml/min/kg (76%)	>80% predicted
VO_2 at AT	10.8 ml/min/kg (66%)	>40% predicted VO_2 peak
VO_2/WR slope	11.3	9–12 and linear
VO_2/HR – Oxygen pulse	8 ml/beat (91%)	>80% predicted
Peak HR	119 bpm (84%)	>85% predicted
Heart rate reserve	23%	<20%
Heart rate recovery	10% peak HR at 1 minute	>10% peak HR at 1 minute
$VEVCO_2$ (at AT/ slope)	38	<32
Breathing reserve	31%	>30%
SpO_2	>95%	>95%

- Is the mechanism of exercise limitation visible and does it make sense with the clinical picture?
  - Potentially. This test shows reduced cardiopulmonary fitness and is consistent with cardiovascular limitation (although there could be contribution from ventilatory or pulmonary vascular factors).

Example 2

Another typical CPET for a patient with cardiovascular disease is shown in Figures 22.3 and 22.4 and Table 22.2 and described in 'Test Review and Interpretation'.

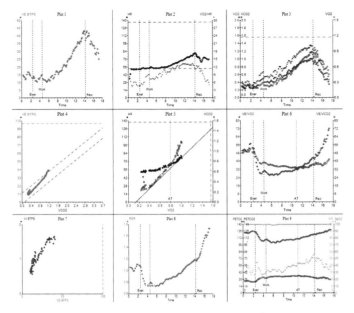

Figure 22.3 Cardiovascular limitation CPET 2: Wasserman plot

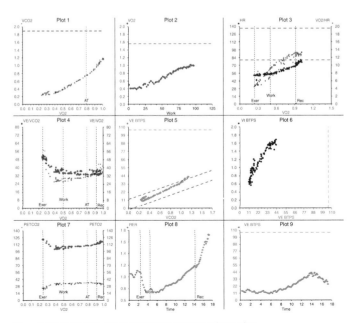

Figure 22.4 Cardiovascular limitation CPET 2: Whipp plot

Table 22.2 Cardiovascular limitation CPET 2 parameters

Exercise parameters	Test result	Normal range
Maximum work	91 watts (97%)	>80% predicted
METS	3.7 (65%)	>80% predicted
RER at peak exercise	1.14	>1.15
Cardiopulmonary Parameters		
Peak VO_2	13.0 ml/min/kg (66%)	>80% predicted
VO_2 at AT	10.1 ml/min/kg (78%)	>40% predicted VO_2 peak
VO_2/WR slope	7.3	9–12 and linear
VO_2/HR – Oxygen pulse	13 ml/beat (118%)	>80% predicted
Peak HR	76 bpm (56%)	>85% predicted
Heart rate reserve	>20%	<20%
Heart rate recovery	>10% peak HR at 1 minute	>10% peak HR at 1minute
$VEVCO_2$ (at AT/slope)	34	<32
Breathing reserve	60%	>30%
SpO_2	>95%	>95%

Test Review and Interpretation

- Was the patient's effort maximal?
  - Uncertain, this test needs to be interpreted with caution. The RER was <1.15 (but is borderline at 1.14), the maximum work rate was >80% predicted but the maximum heart rate was markedly <85% predicted.
- Is the patient's exercise capacity normal?
  - No. Peak VO_2 is reduced, and whilst VO_2/WR gradient is initially normal, there is a reduction/flattening of the gradient at peak workload.

- When does anaerobic metabolism begin?
  - The AT is low in absolute terms, but >40% of the actual VO_2 peak.

- Is circulation or oxygen transport normal?
  - No. Whilst the oxygen pulse is reported as 13 ml/beat (118% of predicted), we need to cross-check other parameters/plots.
  - Whilst heart rate does rise in a linear fashion initially, there is change in the gradient (steepening) of heart rate, which corresponds with the flattening of the oxygen pulse, being suggestive of myocardial ischaemia.
  - Peak HR is only 56% predicted. Hence the oxygen pulse is likely to be artificially inflated due to chronotropic insufficiency.
  - Additionally, the oxygen pulse exhibits a plateau towards peak exercise (with decline seen on the Wasserman plot). This finding is consistent with evolving cardiac ischaemia and reducing pump function. Correlation with the ECG in this case showed developing ischaemic changes. However, CPET is a more sensitive test than ECG in terms of ST changes, and the absence of ST changes does not exclude evolving ischaemia.

- Is ventilation or V/Q matching normal?
  - Partially. SpO_2 and breathing reserve are normal.
  - However, $VEVCO_2$ slope and $VEVCO_2$ at AT are both elevated – in this context it is likely cardiac in origin (due to increased dead space fraction) given the shape of the oxygen pulse and VO_2 curves, but possible contribution from concurrent ventilatory or pulmonary vascular limitation needs to be considered.

- Is the mechanism of exercise limitation visible, and does it make sense with the clinical picture?
  - Yes. This test shows reduced cardiopulmonary fitness, likely secondary to cardiac limitation (potentially with a degree of deconditioning) with chronotropic insufficiency (e.g. beta-blockade, sinus node dysfunction, or diabetes).
  - The acute flattening of the VO_2 work rate slope, with corresponding flattening of the oxygen pulse with a reciprocal increase in the gradient of the heart rate response, is highly

suggestive of myocardial ischaemia with or without ST segment changes.
- ○ This occurs at clinically relevant values and warrants further investigation (e.g. CT angiogram), and management should be considered.

Chapter 23

Ventilatory Limitation

- Patients with ventilatory limitation often have a multifactorial picture. The predominant issue with lung disease is often difficulty clearing carbon dioxide. However, other issues such as diffusion limitation, pulmonary vascular disease, and deconditioning often coexist.

- All patients should have pretest spirometry, which can highlight any obstructive or restrictive patterns before proceeding with an exercise test.

  ○ MVV is calculated from the measured FEV1 (or the predicted values for the patient), and is particularly important to measure this in respiratory patients, otherwise breathing reserve may be overestimated.

- The general parameters that suggest ventilatory limitation include the following:

  ○ Reduced maximum workload

  ○ High resting RER (may be due to hyperventilation or may be normal due to chronic compensatory changes with a low $ETCO_2$)

  ○ Reduced peak VO_2

  ○ AT can be normal/low/not identifiable or absent

  ○ RCP is not usually seen

  ○ Flattened Vt/VE curve

  ○ Low breathing reserve

  ○ Elevated $VEVCO_2$ (at AT and slope)

  ○ Normal or low resting SpO_2 with decline during exercise.

- A typical CPET for a patient with ventilatory limitation is shown in Figures 23.1 and 23.2, and Table 23.1.

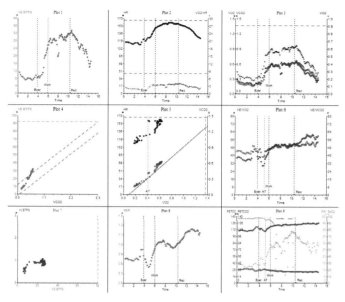

Figure 23.1 Ventilatory limitation CPET: Wasserman plot

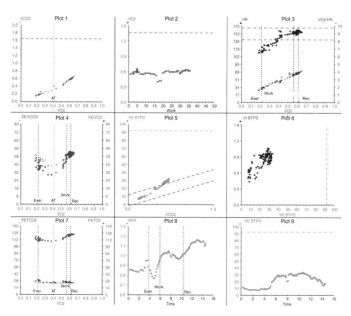

Figure 23.2 Ventilatory limitation CPET: Whipp plot

Table 23.1 Ventilatory limitation CPET – Parameters

Exercise parameters	Test result	Normal range
Maximum work	34 watts (39%)	>80% predicted
METS	3.2 (47%)	>80% predicted
RER at peak exercise	0.99	>1.15
Cardiopulmonary parameters		
Peak VO_2	11.2 ml/min/kg (47%)	>80% predicted
VO_2 at AT	7.1 ml/min/kg (30%)	>40% predicted VO_2 peak
VO_2/WR slope	1.77	9–12 and linear
VO_2/HR – oxygen pulse	4 ml/beat (50%)	>80% predicted
Peak HR	158 bpm (95%)	>85% predicted
Heart rate reserve	<20%	<20%
Heart rate recovery	>10% peak HR at 1 minute	>10% peak HR at 1 minute
$VEVCO_2$ (at AT/slope)	39	<32
Breathing reserve	7%	>30%
SpO_2	Nadir at 94%	>95%

Test Review and Interpretation

- Was the patient's effort maximal?
  - No, this is a submaximal test. The RER was <1.15, the maximum work rate was <80% predicted; however, the maximum heart rate was >85% predicted.
- Is the patient's exercise capacity normal?
  - No, peak VO_2 is <80% predicted with a flat trajectory, and VO_2/WR slope is markedly low.

- When does anaerobic metabolism begin?
  - The AT is low in absolute terms and being <40% of the predicted VO_2.
- Is circulation or oxygen transport normal?
  - In part. Peak HR, HR reserve, and HR recovery are all within normal limits.
  - However, the oxygen pulse is low with a flat but rising trajectory.
  - $VEVCO_2$ is elevated. With normal cardiovascular parameters, this needs review with ventilatory and gas exchange parameters.
- Is ventilation or V/Q matching normal?
  - No. SpO_2 has dropped below 95% and $VEVCO_2$ is elevated, both of which may indicate a degree of pulmonary vascular limitation.
  - Usually, in patients with lung disease we expect the VEmax to be >70% predicted (with a breathing reserve of <30%). In this test however, the VEmax for the test is markedly below the predicted value at 32.3 L. In such cases it can be helpful to calculate the MVV.
  - $(MVV = FEV1 \times 40)$.
  - This patient's FEV1 was 0.87 L, resulting in an MVV of 34.8 L and a markedly reduced breathing reserve of 7%.
- Is the mechanism of exercise limitation visible, and does it make sense with the clinical picture?
  - Yes. This test shows reduced cardiopulmonary fitness with the primary cause being ventilatory limitation (with potential for concurrent pulmonary vascular limitation). These results need correlation with pretest spirometry, which may show evidence of an obstructive or restrictive pattern.

Pulmonary Vascular Limitation

- Pulmonary hypertension causes can be classified as in Table 24.1.
- The underlying principles is that whilst ventilation may be unaffected, the pulmonary vascular system cannot accommodate the increase in blood flow seen during exercise, and as such cardiac output is low.

Table 24.1 Classification of pulmonary hypertension

Classification	Examples can include
Pulmonary arterial hypertension	• Idiopathic • Inherited • Drug/toxin or radiation related • Associated conditions, for example connective tissue disorders, HIV, and portal hypertension • Pulmonary veno-occlusive disease • Pulmonary capillary haemangiomatosis
Due to left heart disease	• Left ventricular dysfunction (systolic/diastolic) • Valvular disease and inflow/outflow obstruction • Congenital heart disease
Due to Lung disease and/or hypoxia	• Chronic obstructive pulmonary disease • Interstitial lung disease • Sleep-disordered breathing
Due to chronic thromboembolic disease or pulmonary arterial occlusion	• Chronic pulmonary emboli • Angiosarcoma and intravascular tumours • Arteritis
Unclear and/or multifactorial mechanisms	• Haematological disorders, for example splenectomy • Systemic disorders, for example sarcoidosis • Metabolic disorders, for example thyroid disease • Other, for example chronic renal failure

- Typical CPET findings in pulmonary vascular limitation include the following:
  - Reduced peak VO_2
  - Low or reduced AT (<40% predicted peak VO_2)
  - Reduced oxygen pulse, which may plateau
  - Elevated VEVCO$_2$
  - Falling SpO$_2$ during exercise.

A typical for a patient with pulmonary vascular limitation is shown in Figures 24.1 and 24.2 and Table 24.2.

Test Review and Interpretation

- Was the patient's effort maximal?
  - No, this was a submaximal test. The RER was <1.15, the maximum work rate was <80% predicted, and the maximum heart rate was <85% predicted.

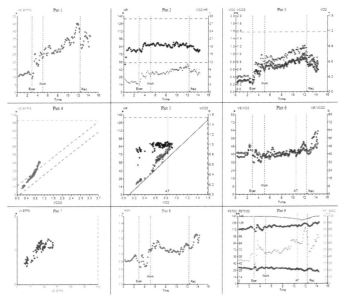

Figure 24.1 Pulmonary vascular limitation CPET: Wasserman plot

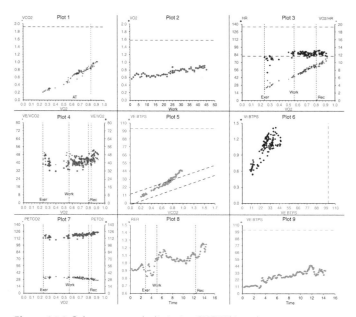

Figure 24.2 Pulmonary vascular limitation CPET: Whipp plot

- Is the patient's exercise capacity normal?
  - No. Peak VO_2 is <80% predicted and VO_2/WR slope is low.
- When does anaerobic metabolism begin?
  - The AT may have just been reached, but is low in absolute terms whilst being >40% of the predicted peak VO_2.
- Is circulation or oxygen transport normal?
  - Mostly. Peak HR is lower than <85 (this patient was receiving treatment with beta-blockers), whilst HR reserve and oxygen pulse are all normal. HR recovery is borderline.
  - $VEVCO_2$ is elevated. With largely normal cardiovascular parameters, this needs review with ventilatory and gas exchange parameters.
- Is ventilation or V/Q matching normal?
  - No. SpO_2 has fallen to a nadir of 93% towards peak exercise and there is an elevated $VEVCO_2$. Breathing reserve is normal (which reduces the likelihood of ventilatory limitation).

Table 24.2 Pulmonary vascular limitation CPET parameters

Exercise parameters	Test result	Normal range
Maximum work	44 watts (52%)	>80% predicted
METS	2.6 (58%)	>80% predicted
RER at peak exercise	1.11	>1.15
Cardiopulmonary parameters		
Peak VO_2	9.2 ml/min/kg (58%)	>80% predicted
VO_2 at AT	8.4 ml/min/kg (52%)	>40% predicted VO_2 peak
VO_2/WR slope	7.9	9–12 and linear
VO_2/HR – oxygen pulse	11 ml/beat (96%)	>80% predicted
Peak HR	82 bpm (61%)	>85% predicted
Heart rate reserve	>20%	<20%
Heart rate recovery	10% peak HR at 1 minute	>10% peak HR at 1 minute
$VEVCO_2$ (at AT/ slope)	39	<32
Breathing reserve	51%	>30%
SpO_2	Nadir of 93%	>95%

- Is the mechanism of exercise limitation visible, and does it make sense with the clinical picture?
  - Yes. This test shows reduced cardiopulmonary fitness, and a falling SpO_2 with elevated $VEVCO_2$ is suggestive of pulmonary vascular limitation (often in pulmonary vascular disease the $VEVCO_2$ slope is significantly elevated >40). Further investigation to estimate pulmonary pressures is warranted (e.g. transthoracic echocardiogram or CTPA).

Chapter 25

Peripheral Vascular Limitation

- Peripheral vascular disease can affect the arterial and/or venous supply to the lower limbs. As such, during exercise and times of increased oxygen demand, the diseased vessels can limit the flow of oxygenated blood to leg muscles. This results in an early anaerobic threshold, build-up of lactic acid, and the onset of claudication, which can result in termination of the test.
- Typical CPET findings in peripheral vascular limitation include the following:
  - Reduced maximum workload
  - Reduced peak VO_2
  - Reduced VO_2/WR slope
  - Low or reduced AT
  - Potentially reduced O_2 pulse (with/without early plateau)
  - High HR reserve
  - High breathing reserve.

A typical CPET for a patient with peripheral vascular limitation is shown in Figures 25.1 and 25.2 and Table 25.1.

Test Review and Interpretation

- Was the patient's effort maximal?
  - No, and therefore needs to be interpreted with caution.
  - The RER is <1.15, which usually indicates a submaximal test. This patient may have terminated the test early due to claudication.
  - Maximal work and maximum heart rate are lower than predicted.

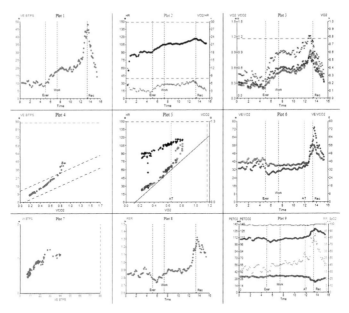

Figure 25.1 Peripheral vascular limitation CPET: Wasserman plot

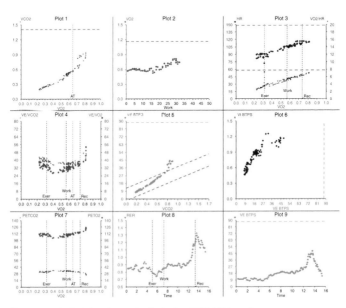

Figure 25.2 Peripheral vascular limitation CPET: Whipp plot

Table 25.1 Peripheral vascular limitation CPET parameters

Exercise parameters	Test result	Normal range
Maximum work	29 watts (47%)	>80% predicted
METS	3.7 (72%)	>80% predicted
RER at peak exercise	1.14	>1.15
Cardiopulmonary parameters		
Peak VO$_2$	12.8 ml/min/kg (72%)	>80% predicted
VO$_2$ at AT	9.9 ml/min/kg (77%)	>40% predicted VO$_2$ peak
VO$_2$/WR slope	7.74	9–12 and linear
VO$_2$/HR – oxygen pulse	7 ml/beat (93%)	>80% predicted
Peak HR	115 bpm (77%)	>85% predicted
Heart rate reserve	>20%	<20%
Heart rate recovery	10% peak HR at 1 minute	>10% peak HR at 1 minute
VEVCO$_2$ (at AT/ slope)	38	<32
Breathing reserve	52%	>30%
SpO$_2$	>95%	>95%

- Is the patient's exercise capacity normal?
  - No, peak VO$_2$ is <80% predicted and the VO$_2$/WR slope is low.
- When does anaerobic metabolism begin?
  - The AT is low in absolute terms, whilst being at >40% of the predicted and actual VO$_2$.
- Is circulation or oxygen transport normal?
  - In part. Both the peak HR and oxygen pulse are reduced, whilst HR reserve and HR recovery are normal or near-normal. This is possibly in keeping with early test termination.

- ○ The $VEVCO_2$, however, are elevated at 38, which may indicate cardiovascular disease, but requires correlation with ventilatory plots and SpO_2.

- Is ventilation or V/Q matching normal?

  - ○ Mostly. Breathing reserve and SpO_2 are both normal.
  - ○ $VEVCO_2$ is elevated at 38, suggesting ventilator inefficiency. It may also indicate cardiovascular or pulmonary vascular limitation.
  - ○ Additionally, there is evidence of hyperventilation at peak exercise. The increased in VE seen on Vt versus VE slope is mostly from increased RR, as Vt is limited to around 1 litre. This suggests a degree of airflow obstruction and should be corroborated with the FEV1 from pretest spirometry.

- Is the mechanism of exercise limitation visible, and does it make sense with the clinical picture?

  - ○ It is likely that there is more than one mechanism of exercise limitation at play. The overall picture with raised ventilator equivalents suggests potential for smoking-related lung disease with peripheral vascular limitation with or without a degree of deconditioning.

Peripheral Muscle Limitation

Chapter

26

- Oxidative phosphorylation supplies the majority of the ATP required to match the energy needs of skeletal muscle during exercise.
- Several disorders (including chemotherapy) can interfere with muscle metabolism or mitochondrial function, causing exercise limitation. They can be categorised as follows:
  - Glycogenolysis and glycolysis disorders (e.g. McArdle Disease)
  - Mitochondrial myopathies (e.g. MELAS syndrome)
  - Lipid metabolism disorders (although the changes seen during CPET for these disorders are relatively minor).
- These patients may benefit from peri-procedural blood sampling to measure lactate, ammonia, and creatine kinase.
- Typical CPET findings in peripheral muscle limitation include the following:
  - Reduced maximum workload
  - RER can be low throughout exercise (glycogenolysis/glycolysis disorders) or very high (mitochondrial myopathies)
  - Reduced peak VO_2
  - Potentially elevated VO_2/WR slope (glycogenolysis/glycolysis disorders)
  - Absent or low AT
  - Reduced O_2 pulse (with/without early plateau)
  - Rapid early rise in HR
  - Potentially elevated $VEVO_2$ (mitochondrial myopathies)
  - Normal or elevated $VEVCO_2$ with normal or low $PETCO_2$
  - Reduced OUES.

A typical CPET for a patient with peripheral muscle limitation is shown in Figures 26.1 and 26.2 and Table 26.1.

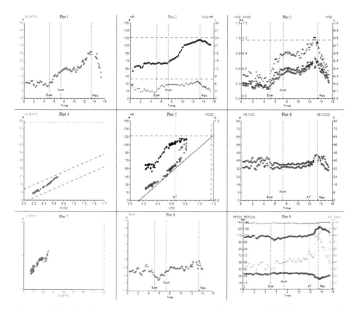

Figure 26.1 Peripheral muscle and mitochondrial limitation CPET: Wasserman plot

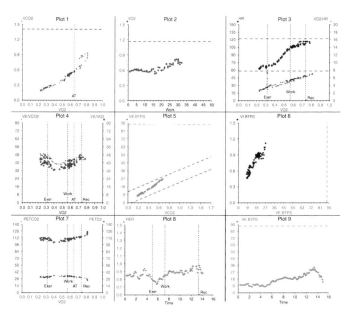

Figure 26.2 Peripheral muscle and mitochondrial limitation CPET: Whipp plot

Table 26.1 Peripheral muscle and mitochondrial limitation CPET parameters

Exercise parameters	Test result	Normal range
Maximum work	34 watts (51%)	>80% predicted
METS	3.9 (74%)	>80% predicted
RER at peak exercise	0.99	>1.15
Cardiopulmonary parameters		
Peak VO_2	12.8 ml/min/kg (72%)	>80% predicted
VO_2 at AT	No AT	>40% predicted VO_2 peak
VO_2/WR slope	9.0	9–12 and linear
VO_2/HR – oxygen pulse	7.5 ml/beat (60%)	>80% predicted
Peak HR	118 bpm (94%)	>85% predicted
Heart rate reserve	<20%	<20%
Heart rate recovery	>10% peak HR at 1 minute	>10% peak HR at 1 minute
$VEVCO_2$ (at AT/slope)	34	<32
$VEVO_2$	32	20–30
Breathing reserve	42%	>30%
SpO_2	>95%	>95%

Test Review and Interpretation

- Was the patient's effort maximal?
  - Needs to be interpreted with caution.
  - RER is <1.15; however, looking at panel 3 on the Wasserman plot, we can see that VCO_2 does not exceed VO_2 at any point. Hence RER cannot rise above 1.0.
  - Maximum work is <80%, whilst maximum HR is >85%.
- Is the patient's exercise capacity normal?

- ○ No. Both peak VO_2 is <80% predicted and VO_2/WR slope is at the low end of the normal range.
- When does anaerobic metabolism begin?
  - ○ There is no anaerobic threshold.
- Is circulation or oxygen transport normal?
  - ○ Mostly. Oxygen pulse is below the lower end of normal, and <80% predicted. Otherwise, peak HR, HR reserve, and HR recovery are normal.
  - ○ $VEVCO_2$ is mildly elevated.
  - ○ Note the early rapid rise in HR.
- Is ventilation or V/Q matching normal?
  - ○ Mostly. Breathing reserve and SpO_2 are both normal, and $VEVCO_2$ is mildly elevated.
  - ○ Note that the $VEVO_2$ is mildly elevated at 32.
- Is the mechanism of exercise limitation visible, and does it make sense with the clinical picture?
  - ○ The reduced RER, peak VO_2, absence of an AT with reduced oxygen pulse, and elevated $VEVO_2$ but with otherwise relatively normal cardiovascular and ventilatory/gas exchange parameters implies exercise limitation is muscular in origin (e.g. McArdle disease).

CPET and Dyspnoea

CPET is a useful tool in the assessment of unexplained dyspnoea, and is increasingly being used to investigate the underlying cause. In order to better understand how CPET can be used in this manner, we will spend some time exploring dyspnoea.

What Is Dyspnoea?

- Dyspnoea is a subjective symptom which describes an awareness of discomfort related to breathing.
- There are synonymous terms, including 'breathlessness' and 'shortness of breath'.
- The term encompasses a number of different sensations that a patient might experience, including the following:
  - Increased work/effort to breath
  - Tightness when breathing
  - Air hunger (a sensation of 'not getting enough air').
- The pathophysiology of dyspnoea is complex.
- Dyspnoea can be physiological, pathophysiological, or psychological in origin.
- It is an important predictor of exercise tolerance, quality of life, and mortality.

Physiology of Dyspnoea

- Ordinarily, breathing is an unconscious process in which the sensory information associated with breathing is 'filtered' from the central nervous system (reducing the processing of 'unnecessary' sensory information).
- However, there is a volitional element which allows humans to 'become aware' of their breathing, and a 'gating process' involved in respiratory monitoring.

- The patient's experience of dyspnoea is multifaceted and the neurophysiology of dyspnoea is not fully understood.
- Often there will be a physiological impairment that impairs homeostasis, leading to stimulation of pulmonary and extrapulmonary afferent receptors, which relay inputs to the cerebral cortex.
- After being processed in the cerebral cortex, when dyspnoea is 'perceived', a patient will ascribe meaning to the symptom. Depending on the context, this may be normal (e.g. after exercise), or potentially unpleasant or threatening (e.g. in disease processes).
- In essence, there are two broad processes that can cause dyspnoea:
  - A physiological or pathophysiological process that results in activation of sensory afferents (e.g. respiratory, cardiovascular, or neuro-muscular pathology)
  - A psychological affective process in which the sensation, having been perceived, is regarded as unpleasant and/or threatening.
- There are multiple stimuli that can activate respiratory afferents. Figure 27.1 shows a schematic representation of the various stimuli, receptors, and pathways involved in the control of breathing and processing of dyspnoea.

Dyspnoea Sensations

- Different physiological mechanisms cause the sensations of dyspnoea.
- It is possible that these mechanisms operate in parallel and can vary in intensity.
- Air hunger
  - Frequently this is the most unpleasant sensation of dyspnoea.
  - Thought be the result of either or both of the following mechanisms:
    - Increased stimulation of central chemoreceptors in the brainstem (especially in the presence of hypoxia or hypercapnia).
    - Inadequate ventilatory response.
- Increased effort or work of breathing
  - Usually, the result is one of the following two factors:

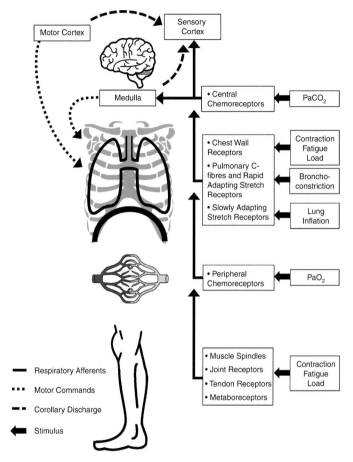

Figure 27.1 Schematic of the control of breathing and processing of dyspnoea

- Increased impedance to breathing (e.g. increased resistance or reduced lung/chest wall compliance) with increased muscle load
- Respiratory muscle fatigue/weakness.
    ○ It is likely to be the result of the following:
    ○ Stimulation of sensory afferents in respiratory muscles

- ◦ Increased awareness of outgoing voluntary motor command (involving the motor cortex and potentially the medulla – so-called corollary discharge).
- Tightness
  - ◦ The sensation of chest tightness is not necessarily attributable to the sensation of work of breathing.
  - ◦ It is thought to be the result of bronchoconstriction as a result of stimulation of airway receptors and pulmonary afferents.

Dyspnoea and Exercise

- Exercise results in increased exertion, both in terms of limb muscles and from the respiratory system.
- As we have established, breathing is closely aligned with increasing muscular activity and cardiovascular demands.
- In normal, healthy subjects, it is unusual for dyspnoea to be the cause of exercise limitation (the primary cause is usually muscular fatigue).
  - ◦ An exception to this can be exercise-induced bronchoconstriction.
- Dyspnoea is a common cause of limitation in patients with cardiopulmonary disease and may be due to several physiological mechanisms, for example:
  - ◦ Dynamic hyperinflation leading to airflow obstruction
  - ◦ Dynamic hyperinflation leading to vascular obstruction
  - ◦ The effects of hypercapnia.
- In these patients, there is usually a problem matching respiratory motor commands with the respiratory system's muscular response.

Assessing Dyspnoea with CPET

- In a similar manner to pain measurement, intensity of dyspnoea intensity can be measured using various scales. Two scales are validated:
  - ◦ Visual analogue scale (in which intensity of shortness of breath is marked on a line between two extremes), shown in Figure 27.2
  - ◦ Modified Borg scale for dyspnoea, in which dyspnoea is rated on a scale of 1 to 10 at rest and during activity.
- Care must be taken to properly elucidate the exact sensation being experienced (air hunger, increased effort, or tightness).

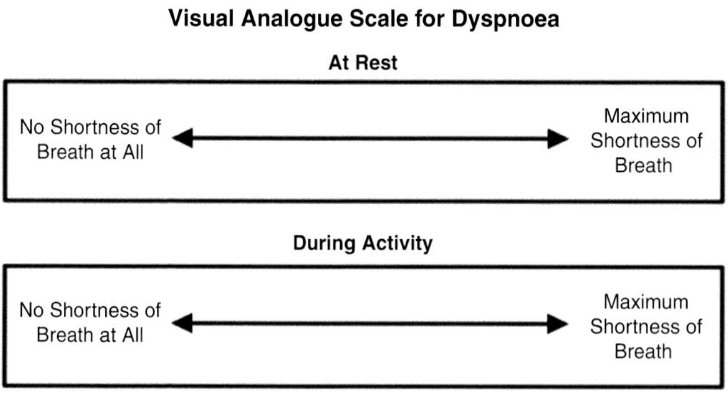

Visual Analogue Scale for Dyspnoea

At Rest

No Shortness of Breath at All	←——————————→	Maximum Shortness of Breath

During Activity

No Shortness of Breath at All	←——————————→	Maximum Shortness of Breath

Figure 27.2 Visual analogue scale for dyspnoea

- Measuring the affective component has proven difficult, although some studies have suggested using the Borg scale and replacing dyspnoea intensity with anxiety.
- No consensus currently exists for which ergometer (treadmill or cycle) is best used to assess dyspnoea.
- The list of potential differential diagnoses for dyspnoea is extensive (see Table 27.1).
- The potential mechanisms of dyspnoea that can be revealed by cardiopulmonary exercise testing include the following:
  - Deconditioning
  - Cardiovascular
  - Ventilatory
  - Pulmonary vascular
  - Peripheral vascular
  - Peripheral muscular (e.g. mitochondrial myopathies)
  - Dysfunctional breathing.
- These will show the same patterns that we see with exercise limitation.
- We will, however, examine dysfunctional breathing in more detail.
- CPET allows for several different mechanisms of dyspnoea to be assessed simultaneously, which we will explore in the next chapter.

Exercise Capacity, Exercise Limitation, and Dyspnoea

Table 27.1 Differential diagnoses of dyspnoea

System	Example pathology
Physiological	<ul><li>Exercise</li><li>Obesity</li><li>Deconditioning</li><li>Pregnancy</li></ul>
Cardiovascular	
• Arrhythmia	• Atrial fibrillation, Sick sinus syndrome, and so on
• Myocardial	• Cardiomyopathy, myocarditis, and so on
• Coronary	• Ischaemia, infarction, and so on
• Valvular	• Stenotic or regurgitant valve
• Pericardial	• Pericarditis, effusion, constriction, and so on
• Congenital	• ASD, Tetralogy of Fallot
• Vascular	• Superior vena cava obstruction
Respiratory	
• Airway	• Tracheomalacia, vocal cord dysfunction, foreign body, and so on
• Obstructive	• Asthma, COPD, bronchiectasis, obstructive sleep apnoea, and so on
• Restrictive	• Interstitial lung disease, sarcoidosis, and so on
• Alveolar	• Pneumonia, aspiration, TB, carcinoma, and so on
• Interstitial	• Drugs (e.g. amiodarone), radiation, lymphangitis
• Pleural	• Effusion, pleuritis, pneumothorax, mesothelioma
• Vascular	• Pulmonary embolus, idiopathic pulmonary hypertension, and so on
Haematological	• Anaemia, methaemoglobinaemia, and so on
Neurological	• Amyotrophic lateral sclerosis, myasthenia gravis, polio, and so on
Psychological	• Anxiety
Muscular	• Mitochondrial myopathy
Metabolic	• Thyroid disease, Cushing's syndrome, and so on
Abdominal	• Ascites, gastro-oesophageal reflux disease, hepatopulmonary syndrome, and so on
Pharmacological	• Drug side effect, anaphylaxis

Chapter 28

Dysfunctional Breathing

- A group of conditions in which there is a change in the normal biomechanical pattern of breathing, which can result in both respiratory and non-respiratory symptoms, but is not due to an organic cause.
- It has been suggested that dysfunctional breathing (DB) can be classified into two broad groups, which have different pathophysiology:
  - Thoracic (may have a physiological or psychological trigger, e.g. exercise, disease, and bereavement)
  - Extra-thoracic (in which the pathophysiology also involves changes of the upper airway, for example laryngomalacia).
- Dysfunctional breathing is not simply hyperventilation. Several different dysfunctional breathing patterns have been described:
  - Hyperventilation syndrome
  - Periodic deep sighing
  - Thoracic dominant breathing (in which breathing mostly utilises the upper thorax with a lack of costal expansion)
  - Forced abdominal expiration (excessive and inappropriate abdominal muscle contraction that aids expiration)
  - Thoraco-abdominal asynchrony (in which there is a delay between rib cage and abdominal contraction).
- CPET is a useful test for identification of DB, especially when a patient's DB is strongly linked to exertion, and may show the following:
  - The key finding is an abnormal erratic breathing pattern in response to exercise.
  - Normal or reduced peak VO_2.

- ○ AT may be normal (although it can be difficult to determine in erratic ventilation).
- ○ VO_2/WR slope is usually within the normal range.
- ○ RER plot may show excessive or erratic variability.
- ○ Normal cardiovascular parameters (peak HR, oxygen pulse, heart rate recovery, etc.).
- ○ The following ventilatory and gas exchange parameters may be seen:
  - ▪ High resting respiratory rate
  - ▪ Respiratory rate increases inappropriately quickly during early exercise (with a near unchanged Vt)
  - ▪ Erratic ventilation with or without frequent sighing
    - • Can be shown with erratic $PETO_2$ a and $PETCO_2$ plots
  - ▪ $VEVCO_2$ slope is usually elevated (>35)
  - ▪ $PETCO_2$ at AT or peak exercise is usually low (<30 mmHg at rest and during exercise)
  - ▪ VD/Vt is usually normal but may be high
  - ▪ A plot of respiratory rate (sometimes called breathing frequency) and tidal volume (Vt) against minute ventilation (VE) can be helpful in identifying erratic breathing patterns (see Figure 28.1).
- Dysfunctional breathing can often be treated with breathing retraining by respiratory physiotherapists.
- A typical CPET for a patient with unexplained dyspnoea is shown in Figures 28.2 and 28.3 and Table 28.1.

Test Review and Interpretation

- Was the patient's effort maximal?
  - ○ Possibly. Whilst RER is >1.15 (with an erratic plot), maximum work is <80% predicted and peak HR is <85% predicted.
  - ○ Of interest, the resting RER (panel 8) is near 1.0, suggesting a degree of anticipatory hyperventilation.
- Is the patient's exercise capacity normal?
  - ○ Yes. Peak VO_2 is >80% predicted and the VO_2/WR slope is normal.
- When does anaerobic metabolism begin?

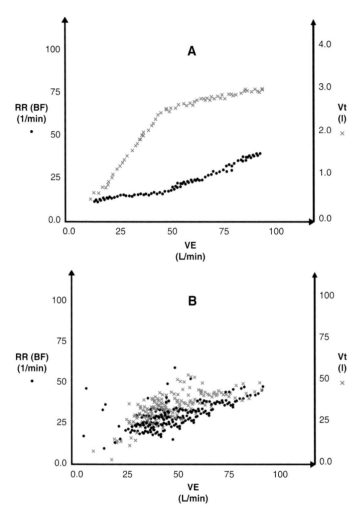

Figure 28.1 Plots of RR (breathing frequency) and tidal volume (Vt) against minute ventilation (VE) in a normal subject (A) and dysfunctional breathing (B)

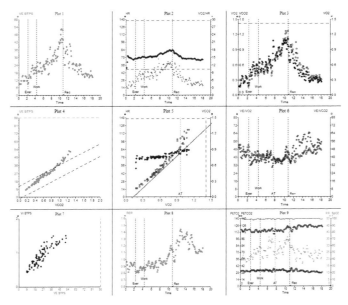

Figure 28.2 Unexplained dyspnoea CPET: Wasserman plot with parameters

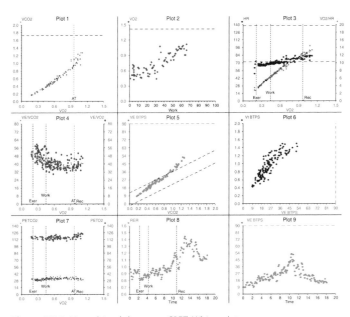

Figure 28.3 Unexplained dyspnoea CPET: Whipp plot

Table 28.1 Unexplained dyspnoea CPET parameters

Exercise parameters	Test result	Normal range
Maximum work	54 watts (68%)	>80% predicted
METS	4.2 (83%)	>80% predicted
RER at peak exercise	1.2	>1.15
Cardiopulmonary parameters		
Peak VO_2	14.8 ml/min/kg (82%)	>80% predicted
VO_2 at AT	12.3 ml/min/kg (83%)	>40% predicted VO_2 peak
VO_2/WR slope	9.7	9–12 and linear
VO_2/HR – oxygen pulse	15 ml/beat (141%)	>80% predicted
Peak HR	80 bpm (58%)	>85 predicted
Heart rate reserve	>20%	<20%
Heart rate recovery	>10% peak HR at 1 minute	>10% peak HR at 1 minute
$VEVCO_2$ (at AT/ slope)	36	<32
Breathing reserve	35%	>30%
SpO_2	>95%	>95%

○ The AT is appropriate in absolute terms and is >40% of the predicted VO_2.

• Is circulation or oxygen transport normal?

○ Not entirely. Peak HR is 58% predicted, suggesting chronotropic insufficiency. This may have artificially elevated the oxygen pulse (which is 141% predicted), and whilst the plot is somewhat erratic it does not show signs of plateau, which is reassuring. Otherwise, HR reserve and HR recovery are normal.

○ $VEVCO_2$ is elevated.

- Is ventilation or V/Q matching normal?
  - Not entirely. Whilst SpO_2 and breathing reserve are all within normal limits, $VEVCO_2$ are elevated with an erratic plot.
  - Of interest, $PETCO_2$ at rest is low (30 mmHg) and at peak exercise is at the low end of normal (35 mmHg).
  - Additionally, it can see a high degree of variability in RR, VE, and Vt during the test.
- Is the mechanism of exercise limitation visible, and does it make sense with the clinical picture?
  - Whilst exercise does not appear to be significantly limited, there are potential signs of dysfunctional/oscillatory breathing on this CPET. Additionally, there are signs of chronotropic insufficiency and ventilator inefficiency.

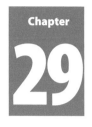

Chapter 29

Peri-operative Risk Stratification and Shared Decision-Making

Increasingly CPET is being used as part of the pre-operative work-up of patients for major surgery. Whilst CPET can not necessarily be used to define a specific risk for a specific patient, it can provide a broad risk stratification which can guide the need for optimisation, prehabilitation, or potential post-operative level of care. It is part of a global assessment of the patient and hard cut-off values should be avoided. A useful mental model is the 'traffic light model' (Figure 29.1).

The use of CPET has been incorporated into several surgical guidelines, although there is variation in terms of the following:

- The parameters which are deemed to confer increased risk
- The threshold values of these parameters
- Surgical specialty and specific operation
- Sensitivity and specificity of each parameter
- The effect of each parameter on mortality, morbidity, length of stay, and so on
- Quality of evidence varies between studies.

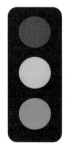

Red Light
- Highest Risk – surgery potentially poses greater a risk to survival than underlying pathology

Amber Light
- Increased Risk – need for increased level of care or to delay surgery for optimisation

Green Light
- Low Risk – can proceed to surgery without delay

Figure 29.1 Traffic light model of peri-operative risk

In general, the following are important parameters:
- Peak VO_2
  - Some guidelines will quote peak VO_2 less than 15 ml/kg/min, which confers higher risk. However, as a specific threshold value it is of limited use when not used for specific surgical procedures.
  - A good rule of thumb is:
    - A low peak VO_2 is associated with higher risk. Risk increases as peak VO_2 gets lower.
    - A peak VO_2 >80% predicted is likely to confer low risk.
- AT
  - The majority of work has studied peri-operative risk related to AT. In general, the following is used:
  - Average risk = AT >10–11 ml/kg/min without evidence of myocardial ischaemia, depending on procedure/data.
  - Higher risk
    - AT >11 ml/kg/min with evidence of myocardial ischaemia
    - AT <11 ml/kg/min.
- $VEVCO_2$
  - Has been shown to be an independent risk factor for morbidity, including peri-operative pulmonary complications and mortality
  - Low risk = $VEVCO_2$ <35
  - Higher risk = $VEVCO_2$ >35
    - In general, the higher the $VEVCO_2$, the higher the risk.

Exercise Prescription

Having found and quantified the degree of exercise limitation by performing a CPET, increasingly peri-operative physicians are prescribing exercise as a form of therapy. Exercise has the additional benefit of not only improving cardiopulmonary fitness, but also reducing morbidity, mortality, and peri-operative risk. Some centres will issue formal exercise prescriptions and will have links with physiotherapists and personal trainers to help facilitate. In terms of general advice, most sources would suggest that individuals should aim for 20–30 minutes of moderate exercise most days of the week. The desired intensity of exercise is often the most difficult to convey to patients, but the following descriptions (with examples) may be helpful:

- Low intensity exercise – you would be able to hold a conversation without pausing for breath (e.g. going for a leisurely walk).
- Moderate intensity – you would start to pause for breath between sentences (e.g. going for a brisk walk).
- High intensity – you would be able to speak a few words, but would need to pause for breath afterwards (e.g. jogging/running).

Shared Decision-Making

Shared decision-making refers to the respectful partnership whereby clinicians and patients make decisions together to help patients make the right choice regarding their condition and treatment options. It is a non-linear process and it is important to identify and consider patient goals and values in addition to the best available evidence and clinical circumstances. It is important to highlight identified patient goals and values in clinic letters.

CPET is one component of the individualised patient risk assessment that feeds into the shared decision-making process. It is not purely about the 'numbers' of CPET, the results need to be contextualised. This may include the use of local outcome data and patient surgical MDT discussions when making decisions about treatments. Help from other speciality colleagues when discussing the available options may be required and knowing where/how they can be accessed is essential.

The '3 talk' model provides a framework to deliver shared decision-making effectively within the CPET clinic and perioperative setting; it is comprised of three separate but interlinking 'talks' outlined next. Whilst some or all of them may be covered in a CPET clinic, it is important to elucidate the patients' goals and vales, as they can underpin further discussions.

- Team talk – in which clinicians and the patient work together, outline the potential options that are available, discuss the patient's goals, and offer support.
- Option talk – in which options are narrowed down, the pros and cons of each are discussed and compared (including no treatment), and risks are communicated.
- Decision talk – where informed preferences are explored and used to make informed decisions.

Further Reading

Part I   What Is Cardiopulmonary Exercise Testing?

- American Thoracic Society; American College of Chest Physicians. ATS/ACCP Statement on cardiopulmonary exercise testing. *Am J Respir Crit Care Med*. 15 January 2003;**167**(2):211–77. https://doi.org/10.1164/rccm.167.2.211. Erratum in: *Am J Respir Crit Care Med*. 15 May 2003;1451–2. PMID: 12524257.
- Carlisle, J and Swart, M. Mid-term survival after abdominal aortic aneurysm. *Br J SUrg*. 2007 Aug; **94**(8):966–92007.
- Fick, A. Uber die Messung des Blutquantums in den Herzventrikeln. *Seitung der Physikalisches und Medicinisches Gesellschaft zu Würzburg*. 1870;**2**:290–1.
- Forman, DE, Myers, J, Lavie, CJ, et al. Cardiopulmonary exercise testing: relevant but underused. *Postgrad Med*. November 2010;**122**(6):68–86. https://doi.org/10.3810/pgm.2010.11.2225. PMID: 21084784; PMCID: PMC9445315.
- Iannetta, D, de Almeida Azevedo, R, Keir, DA, and Murias, JM. Establishing the $\dot{V}o_2$ versus constant-work-rate relationship from ramp-incremental exercise: simple strategies for an unsolved problem. *J Appl Physiol (1985)*. 1 December 2019;**127**(6):1519–27.
- Levett, DZH, Jack, S, Swart, M, et al. Perioperative Exercise Testing and Training Society (POETTS). Perioperative cardiopulmonary exercise testing (CPET): consensus clinical guidelines on indications, organization, conduct, and physiological interpretation. *Br J Anaesth*. March 2018;**120**(3):484–500. https://doi.org/10.1016/j.bja.2017.10.020. Epub 24 November 2017. PMID: 29452805.
- Older, P, Hall, A, and Hader, R. Cardiopulmonary exercise testing as a screening test for perioperative management of major surgery in the elderly. *Chest*. 1999;**116**(2):355–62.
- Older, P, Smith, R, Courtney, P, and Hone, R. Preoperative evaluation of cardiac failure and ischemia in elderly patients by cardiopulmonary exercise testing. *Chest*. 1993;**104**(3):701–4.
- Sietsema K, Sue DY, Stringer WW and Ward S. *Wasserman & Whipp's: Principles of Exercise Testing and Interpretation: Including Pathophysiology and Clinical Applications* Sixth Edition. Wolters Kluwer.
- Snowden, CP, Prentis, JM, Anderson, HL, et al. Submaximal cardiopulmonary exercise testing predicts complications and hospital length of stay in patients undergoing major elective surgery. *Ann Surg*. 2010;**251**:535–41.
- Wilson, BA, Schisler, JC, and Willis, MS. Sir Hans Adolf Krebs: architect of metabolic cycles. *Lab Med*. June 2010;**41**(6):377–80.
- Wilson, R, Davies, S, Yates, D, Redman, J, and Stone, M. Impaired

functional capacity is associated with all-cause mortality after major elective intra-abdominal surgery. *Br J Anaesth.* 2010 Sep;**105**(3):297–303.

• Zhang, XC and Feng, W. Thermodynamic aspects of ATP hydrolysis of actomyosin complex. *Biophys Rep.* 2016;**2**(5):87–94.

Part II   Conducting a Cardiopulmonary Exercise Test

• American Thoracic Society; American College of Chest Physicians. ATS/ACCP Statement on cardiopulmonary exercise testing. *Am J Respir Crit Care Med.* 15 January 2003;**167**(2):211–77. https://doi.org/10.1164/rcc m.167.2.211. Erratum in: *Am J Respir Crit Care Med.* 15 May 2003;1451–2. PMID: 12524257.

• Clinical Management of COVID-19: Living Guideline. World Health Organisation. 23 June 2022. www .who.int/publications-detail-redirect/ WHO-2019-nCoV-clinical-2023.2

• Faghy, MA, Sylvester, KP, Cooper, BG, and Hull, JH. Cardiopulmonary exercise testing in the COVID-19 endemic phase. *Br J Anaesth.* October 2020;**125** (4):447–9. https://doi.org/10.1016/j .bja.2020.06.006. Epub 11 June 2020. PMID: 32571569; PMCID: PMC7287473.

• Forbregd, TR, Aloyseus, MA, Berg, A, and Greve, G. Cardiopulmonary capacity in children during exercise testing: the differences between treadmill and upright and supine cycle ergometry. *Front Physiol.* 29 November 2019;**10**:1440. https:// doi.org/10.3389/fphys.2019.01440. PMID: 31849698; PMCID: PMC6897055.

• Huszczuk, A, Whipp, BJ, and Wasserman, K. A respiratory gas exchange simulator for routine calibration in metabolic studies. *Eur Respir J.* 1990;**3**(4):465–8.

• Jones, NL, Makrides, L, Hitchcock, C, Chypchar, T, and McCartney, N. Normal standards for an incremental progressive cycle ergometer test. *Am Rev Respir Dis.* 1985;**131**(5):700–8.

• Long COVID and Return to Work – What Works? A Position Paper from the Society of Occupational Medicine. August 2022. Long_COV ID_and_Return_to_Work_What_ Works.pdf (som.org.uk)

• Myers, J, Arena, R, Franklin, B, et al. Recommendations for clinical exercise laboratories: a scientific statement from the American Heart Association. *Circulation.* 2009;**119** (24):3144–61.

• Orr, JL, Williamson, P, Anderson, W, et al. Cardiopulmonary exercise testing: arm crank vs cycle ergometry. *Anaesthesia.* May 2013;**68**(5):497– 501. https://doi.org/10.1111/ana e.12195. PMID: 23573845.

• Pritchard, A, Burns, P, Correia, J, et al. ARTP statement on cardiopulmonary exercise testing 2021. *BMJ Open Respir Res.* November 2021;**8**(1):e001121. https://doi.org/10.1136/bmjresp-2 021-001121. PMID: 34782330; PMCID: PMC8593741.

• Quanjer, P, Tammeling GJ, Cotes JE, et al. Lung volumes and forced ventilatory flows: report working party – standardisation of lung function tests. European Community for Steel and Coal. *Eur Respir J.* 1992;**6**(Suppl. 16):5–40.

- Radtke, T, Crook, S, Kaltsakas, G, et al. ERS statement on standardisation of cardiopulmonary exercise testing in chronic lung diseases. *Eur Resp Rev.* December 2019;**28**(154):180101.
- Reeves, T, Bates, S, Sharp, T, et al. Perioperative Exercise Testing and Training Society (POETTS). Cardiopulmonary exercise testing (CPET) in the United Kingdom: a national survey of the structure, conduct, interpretation and funding. *Perioper Med (Lond).* 26 January 2018;**7**:2. https://doi.org/10.1186/s13741-017-0082-3. Erratum in: *Perioper Med (Lond).* 4 May 2018;**7**:8. PMID: 29423173; PMCID: PMC5787286.
- World Physiotherapy Response to COVID-19. Briefing Paper 9 – Safe Rehabilitation Approaches for People Living with Long COVID: Physical Activity and Exercise. World Physiotherapy. June 2021.COVID-19: Briefing papers | World Physiotherapy.
- Wright, SE, Pearce, B, Snowden, CP, Anderson, H, and Wallis, JP. Cardiopulmonary exercise testing before and after blood transfusion: a prospective clinical study. *Br J Anaesth.* 2014;**113**:91–6.

Part III   Interpreting a Cardiopulmonary Exercise Test

- Baba, R, Nagashima, M, Goto, M, et al. Oxygen uptake efficiency slope: A new index of cardiorespiratory functional reserve derived from the relation between oxygen uptake and minute ventilation during incremental exercise. *J Am Coll Cardiol.* 1996;**28**:1567–72.
- Brubaker, PH and Kitzman, DW. Chronotropic incompetence: Causes, consequences, and management. *Circulation.* 2011;**123**:1010–20.
- Chambers, DJ and Wisely, NA. Cardiopulmonary exercise testing: A beginner's guide to the nine-panel plot. *BJA Educ.* May 2019;**19**(5):158–64. https://doi.org/10.1016/j.bja e.2019.01.009. Epub 20 March 2019. PMID: 33456885; PMCID: PMC7807922.
- Dumitrescu, D and Rosenkranz, S. Graphical data display for clinical cardiopulmonary exercise testing. *Ann Am Thorac Soc.* July 2017;**14** (Suppl. 1):S12–S21. https://doi.org/1 0.1513/AnnalsATS.201612-955FR. PMID: 28541745.
- Glaab, T and Taube, C. Practical guide to cardiopulmonary exercise testing in adults. *Respir Res.* 12 January 2022;**23**(1):9. https://doi .org/10.1186/s12931-021-01895-6. PMID: 35022059; PMCID: PMC8754079.
- Hansen, JE, Sue, DY, and Wasserman, K. Predicted values for clinical exercise testing. *Am Rev Respir Dis.* 1984;**129**(2)Pt. 2:S49–55.
- Hollenberg, M and Tager, IB. Oxygen uptake efficiency slope: An index of exercise performance and cardiopulmonary reserve requiring only submaximal exercise. *J Am Coll Cardiol.* 2000;**36**:194–201.
- Older, P. Anaerobic threshold, is it a magic number to determine fitness for surgery? *Perioper Med (Lond).* 21 February 2013;**2**(1):2. https://doi.or g/10.1186/2047-0525-2-2. PMID: 24472514; PMCID: PMC3964343.
- Sietsema, K, Sue, DY, Stringer, WW, and Ward, S. *Wasserman & Whipp's Principles of Exercise Testing and Interpretation: Including Pathophysiology and Clinical*

Applications, 6th ed. 2020. Wolters Kluwer.

- Wasserman, K, Beaver, WL, and Whipp, BJ. Gas exchange theory and the lactic acidosis (anaerobic) threshold. *Circulation.* 1990;**81** (Suppl. 1):II14–II30.
- Whipp, BJ, Ward, SA, and Wasserman, K. Respiratory markers of the anaerobic threshold. *Adv Cardiol.* 1986;**35**:47–64.

Part IV Assessment of Exercise Capacity and Causes of Exercise Limitation and Dyspnoea

- Barker, N and Everard, ML. Getting to grips with 'dysfunctional breathing'. *Paediatr. Respir. Rev.* 2015;**16**:53–61. https://doi.org/10.10 16/j.prrv.2014.10.001.
- Borg, GA. Psychophysical bases of perceived exertion. *Med Sci Sports Exerc.* 1982;**14**:377–81.
- Boulding, R, Stacey R, Niven R and Fowler SJ Dysfunctional breathing: A review of the literature and proposal for classification. *European Respiratory Review.* September 2016;**25**(141):287–94.
- Brunelli, A, Charloux, A, Bolliger, CT, et al. European Respiratory Society and European Society of Thoracic Surgeons joint task force on fitness for radical therapy. ERS/ESTS clinical guidelines on fitness for radical therapy in lung cancer patients (surgery and chemo-radiotherapy). *Eur Respir J.* July 2009;**34**(1):17–41. https://d oi.org/10.1183/09031936.0018430 8. Erratum in: Eur Respir J. September 2009;34(3):782. PMID: 19567600.
- Brunelli, A, Kim, AW, Berger, KI, and Addrizzo-Harris, DJ. Physiologic evaluation of the patient with lung cancer being considered for resectional surgery: Diagnosis and management of lung cancer, 3rd ed.: American College of Chest Physicians evidence-based clinical practice guidelines. *Chest.* May 2013;**143**(Suppl. 5):e166S–e190S. https://doi.org/10.1378/chest .12-2395. Erratum in: Chest. February 2014;145(2):437. PMID: 23649437.
- Ferguson, M and Shulman, M. Cardiopulmonary exercise testing and other tests of functional capacity. *Curr Anesthesiol Rep.* 2022;**12**(1):26–33.
- Guazzi, M, Adams, V, Conraads, V, et al. EACPR/AHA joint scientific statement: Clinical recommendations for cardiopulmonary exercise testing data assessment in specific patient populations. *Eur Heart J.* December 2012;**33**(23):2917–27. https://doi.org/10.1093/eurheartj/ ehs221. Epub 5 September 2012. PMID: 22952138.
- Kothmann, E, Batterham, AM, Owen, SJ, et al. Effect of short-term exercise training on aerobic fitness in patients with abdominal aortic aneurysms: A pilot study. *Br J Anaesth.* 2009;**103**(4):505–10.
- Lim, E, Baldwin, D, Beckles, M, et al. British Thoracic Society; Society for Cardiothoracic Surgery in Great Britain and Ireland. Guidelines on the radical management of patients with lung cancer. *Thorax.* October 2010;**65**(Suppl. 3):iii1–iii27. https:// doi.org/10.1136/thx.2010.145938. PMID: 20940263.

Further Reading

- Mahler, DA and Horowitz, MB. Perception of breathlessness during exercise in patients with respiratory disease. *Med Sci Sports Exerc.* September 1994;**26**(9):1078–81. PMID: 7808239.
- Older, PO and Levett, DZH. Cardiopulmonary exercise testing and surgery. *Ann Am Thorac Soc.* July 2017;**14**(Suppl. 1):S74–S83. https://doi.org/10.1513/AnnalsATS.201610-780.
- Parshall, MB, Schwartzstein, RM, Adams, L, et al. American Thoracic Society Committee on Dyspnea. An official American Thoracic Society statement: Update on the mechanisms, assessment, and management of dyspnea. *Am J Respir Crit Care Med.* 15 February 2012;**185**(4):435–52.
- Richardson, K, Levett, DZH, and Jack, S. Grocott fit for surgery? Perspectives on preoperative exercise testing and training. *Br J Anaesth.* 2017;**119**:34–43.
- Schonborn, JL and Anderson, H. Perioperative medicine: A changing model of care. *BJA Education.* 2019;**19**(1):27–33.
- Snowden, CP, Prentis, JM, Anderson, HL, et al. Submaximal cardiopulmonary exercise testing predicts complications and hospital length of stay in patients undergoing major elective surgery. *Ann Surg.* 2010;**251**(3):535–41.
- Vidotto, LS, Carvalho, CRF, Harvey, A, and Jones, M. Dysfunctional breathing: What do we know? *J Bras Pneumol.* 11 February 2019;**45**(1):e20170347. https://doi.org/10.1590/1806-3713/e20170347. PMID: 30758427; PMCID: PMC6534396.
- Wilson, RC and Jones, PW. A comparison of the visual analogue scale and modified Borg scale for the measurement of dyspnoea during exercise. *Clin Sci (Lond).* 1989;**76**:277–82.

Index

Printed in the United States
by Baker & Taylor Publisher Services